Critical Perspectives
on Health

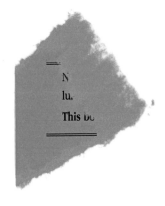

N
lu.
This bo

Also by this author

Cribb, A. and Duncan, P. (2002) *Health Promotion and Professional Ethics*, Oxford: Blackwell Publishing

Critical Perspectives on Health

Peter Duncan

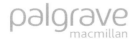

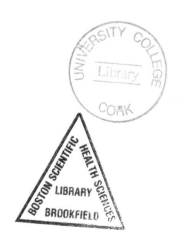

First published in 2007 by
PALGRAVE MACMILLAN
Houndmills, Basingstoke, Hampshire RG21 6XS and
175 Fifth Avenue, New York, N.Y. 10010
Companies and representatives throughout the world

PALGRAVE MACMILLAN is the global academic imprint of the Palgrave
Macmillan division of St. Martin's Press, LLC and of Palgrave Macmillan Ltd.
Macmillan® is a registered trademark in the United States, United Kingdom
and other countries. Palgrave is a registered trademark in the European
Union and other countries.

ISBN-13: 978–1–4039–9452–3
ISBN-10: 1–4039–9452–8

This book is printed on paper suitable for recycling and made from fully
managed and sustained forest sources.

A catalogue record for this book is available from the British Library.

10 9 8 7 6 5 4 3 2 1
16 15 14 13 12 11 10 09 08 07

Printed and bound in China

Contents

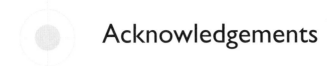

Acknowledgements

I would like to thank my colleagues both in the School of Social Science and Public Policy and the Department of Education and Professional Studies, King's College London who allowed me the time to write this book. I am especially grateful for a period of sabbatical leave during Summer Term 2005 and for the help given by Alan Cribb and Margaret Sills in making this work. I would also like to thank Lynda Thompson at Palgrave Macmillan for her help and support.

The figure that appears on pages 81 and 129 is reproduced by kind permission of Sylvina Tate, School of Integrated Health, University of Westminster; and the Higher Education Academy-Health Science and Practice Subject Centre.

In a year of lots of downs and very few ups, Jane gave me a huge amount of support. So this is for her, and for the girls.

Preface

The idea for this book grew out of my work with students on a range of health studies-related courses and programmes at advanced undergraduate, as well as postgraduate, level. In discussions, it seemed more and more to me that students engaged in these kinds of courses were being presented with enormous challenges. In the first place, they were encountering and having to deal with a range of academic disciplines, each of which claimed to have something important to say about 'health' and about the nature of 'work for health'. Second, they were having to relate these so-called discourses to what, often, they had already understood about 'health' and 'health care' through lengthy periods training and working as professionals in health-related occupations such as nursing. Third, they were being expected to work out new and different ways of thinking about 'health' through drawing together their professional experiences and their developing academic understanding, using in particular processes of 'critical analysis' and 'critical reflection'. These processes were often referred to but never explicitly discussed. Students *just were* expected it seemed, to engage in analysis and reflection as a matter of course.

It appeared to me that each of these three challenges was major in itself. Together, they presented a vast and difficult terrain for people who were very often juggling study with other commitments, both work and personal. In my talks with the students I was working with, I began to develop a conception of the essential 'difficulty of health studies'. Centred on the fundamentally problematic question, 'What is health?' the difficulty seemed to spread out to a range of issues related to dealing with past occupational and professional histories, coping with competing academic and theoretical conceptions and mastering the elusive (but nevertheless taken for granted) skills of analysis and reflection.

I thought that there would be worth in developing an account of 'the difficulty of health studies', engaging in more detailed discussion of the supposed resources available that might help meet the difficulty and trying to apply these to competing academic perspectives on the nature of health. In other words, I wanted to create an account and exploration of the three challenges that seemed to be facing the students I was working with. In doing so, I thought it might be possible to move towards greater understanding of the 'What is health?' question that dominates the field of health studies, and lies at the centre of 'the difficulty of health studies'.

I equally feel a strong sense of perplexity in my work on health studies. So while the idea for this book grew out of conversations with students who were facing the difficulties I've described above, writing it has also been an enormous opportunity to become clearer *myself* about the problems that we face in studying health!

The book is divided into three parts:

Part I: Professional Experience, Academic Study and Health

The beginning three chapters in this first part of the book develop an account of the nature of studying health and, in particular, why 'the difficulty of health studies' is so fundamental. My argument is that the nature of 'health' is vehemently disputed and disagreed about in the first place (Chapter 1). But the roots of this dispute lie at least partly in the conceptions of health that we develop as a result of our health care professional training and experience (Chapter 2). The difficulty is compounded still more by the potential confusion contained within the separate discourses of the academic disciplines (for example, philosophy and sociology) that claim to be telling us important things about 'health'. Moreover, in the interdisciplinary *field* of health studies, we often have to juggle between these disciplines (Chapter 3). The last chapter in this part of the book (Chapter 4) tries to gather these separate components of 'the difficulty of health studies' together and create an agenda for tackling the difficulty. This agenda centres around the need to develop our critical skills (of analysis and reflection) and to apply these to thinking about what the academic disciplines connected to the study of health actually have to say.

Part II: Developing Critical Perspectives

This part of the book sets out ways in which we can develop our skills of critical analysis (Chapter 5) and critical reflection (Chapter 6) to support our study of health. We need both kinds of skills when we engage in health studies. Critical *analysis* is needed in order to dissect the wide range and variety of supposedly rational arguments that are used by academics in support of their discourses on health. We need the capacity to critically *reflect* because ideologies, beliefs and values drive a good deal in these arguments (and our reaction to them). Critical reflection is a process that can support understanding of our emotional and affective reaction to argument and experience.

The Structure of the Book *continued*

Part III: Critical Perspectives on Health

This part of the book uses the understanding that has been developed so far with regard to 'the difficulty of health studies' and the skills required to support us in dealing with this and applies it to try and illuminate a number of health-related academic discourses. Chapter 7 examines discourses from philosophy on the *nature* of health. Chapter 8 considers material that has emerged from ethics that has attempted to establish the kind of *value* that health is and has. In Chapter 9, I look at sociological discourses connected to how health is *produced* and where power in that production might lie. The final chapter of the book (Chapter 10) draws its arguments together and suggests how it might be possible to continue using this experience of dealing with 'the difficulty of health studies', and so developing critical perspectives on health, in both our academic study and our professional lives.

A 'quick reference' glossary of key terms appears after the final chapter, making it easier for readers to understand and navigate their way through the language used by others (as well as within this book!) in the development of critical perspectives.

Thinking points appear often within chapters. They have been designed to help you extend or reflect on your thinking as you make your way through the book's content.

Turning points appear at the end of almost every chapter. Their purpose is to encourage you to think again, and possibly think in new ways, about the material contained in the chapter. Their aim is to encourage you to consider that the discussion and argument within the chapter, no matter how convincing, can always be seen differently. In this way, I hope that they become representative of a reflective approach within the book as a whole; in the field of health studies nothing can be taken for granted – this idea needs to be one of our touchstones as we engage in study.

While the parts of the book connect with each other, and the arguments for both the nature of 'the difficulty of health studies' and how we deal with it are incremental, there is no reason why separate parts and chapters can't be used on their own. If you were interested in a particular issue – for example, the relationship between professional values and beliefs about health – then I would encourage you to concentrate on the relevant sections of the book. Equally, though, I hope you will think there is worth in an extended discussion and debate on the challenge of gaining truly critical perspectives on health!

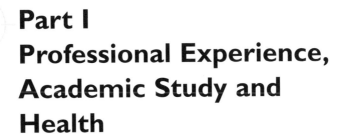

Part I
Professional Experience, Academic Study and Health

1 Studying Health: The Nature of Health and Health-Related Knowledge

What is this chapter going to do?

This chapter begins an argument for why the study of health is complex – an argument that aims ultimately to understand more fully (and so to be better able to deal with) what I will call 'the difficulty of health studies'. This part of the argument is about how dispute on the nature of health itself and disagreement on what we can know about it feed this difficulty. I examine two broad positions on the nature of health: one that it is an objective state; and the other that it depends on peoples' own understanding and interpretation. I argue that both positions cause problems for health studies students. And a 'middle way' out of the difficulty (health can be understood as involving both objective and interpretive elements) is not necessarily a realistic option for the student of health.

Approaching Health Studies

This book is about studying health, and about some of the difficulties involved in such study. But it is also about the enormous possibilities and satisfactions that emerge from careful examination of a highly elusive concept, one that has perplexed and intrigued thinkers, policymakers and practitioners through history and into our own times. A central contention of this book is that recognising, approaching and confronting what I will call 'the difficulty of health studies' leads to the rewards attached to greater understanding – and these rewards benefit personal and professional lives.

So in the first part of this book, I do two main things:

▸ *I describe and discuss the nature of 'the difficulty of health studies'.*
▸ *I start to establish how it might be possible to deal with this difficulty.*

At least some of the fundamental questions connected to the study of health will probably be familiar enough to you already. What is health? What is the nature of the relationship between individuals, society and levels of health (or disease)? What can be done to improve health? How can the wide range of occupations, professions and disciplines involved in the fields of health and health care contribute to 'more health'?

One of the puzzles connected to the study of health is that it sometimes seems as if the more thought that is applied (considering, for example, these kinds of questions), the murkier the territory becomes. Perhaps this is so with the study of almost anything – it may well be true – but I believe that there are particular reasons for this puzzle of 'the more you think about it, the harder it becomes' in the case of health studies.

There are three central stages in my argument for the difficulty of studying health:

▸ In the first place, separate ways of trying to understand the nature of health itself lead in turn to different and conflicting attempts to stake claims about what we can know about health – and how we can know it. (This part of my argument is developed in this first chapter.)

▸ Second, our own occupational or professional identities shape our beliefs about health – and make it much harder for us reasonably to consider alternative perspectives on health. (This part of my argument is considered in Chapter 2.)

▸ Third, the academic disciplines that are supposed to help us in our study of health themselves contribute to misunderstanding and dispute. (I develop this part of my argument in Chapter 3.)

If there was only difficulty in studying health, it would be reasonable to ask what the point of it all was. But I want also to argue that if we think closely and carefully about 'the difficulty of health studies' we ultimately strengthen our ability to engage in work related to health care and health improvement. So Part 1 of this book ends, in Chapter 4, with what might be called an 'agenda' for tackling 'the difficulty of health studies' – an agenda that has emerged from thinking about the nature of the difficulty itself. This is the agenda that is pursued in the remaining parts of the book.

My claim is that 'health' is a problematic field of study. If this is so, then there is a need to think seriously about engaging in it. Construct your own argument for why the study of health is important to you, professionally and/ or personally. What arguments might there be *against* engaging in health studies? How could these be overcome?

Health and the Nature of Knowledge about Health

In the first part of my argument for the difficulty in studying health, I want to approach two questions that are key to health studies:

▶ What can we know about health?
▶ How can we know what we do about it?

These questions have elicited many different kinds of responses on the part of theorists and professionals, not to mention lay people. Responses are frequently conflicting and confusing, and there is a pressing need to try and untangle them if we are to move forward in the study of health.

In theoretical terms, these questions are *epistemological* ones; that is to say, they are questions about the grounds of our knowledge (Lacey, 1976). The two questions are also closely connected. Our decisions about the methods we believe should be employed in order to investigate health issues (*how* can we know what we do about health?) will depend on the way in which we have chosen to answer the question about *what* we can know.

Preceding these epistemological questions, though, are *ontological* ones. Ontological questions are about the existence of something in the first place, aside from questions about how and what we can know of that thing (Lacey, 1976). So in the case of health we would want to ask:

▶ What is the nature of this thing that exists, which is called 'health'?

Or we might even feel the need to ask:

▶ Does 'health' exist in the first place?

The first kind of ontological question seems much more relevant to me than the second sort. It would be hard to imagine the point of trying to argue for or against the very existence of something in the world that we call 'health'. After all, structures have been established, legislation has been enacted, occupations and professions have been founded, in order to address the issue of 'health'. In the United Kingdom (UK), there is a Department of Health, and a National Health Service. There are hospitals, doctors, allied health professions, primary health care systems, environmental health departments and public health intervention programmes. Given all this, how can we reasonably argue against the existence of something called 'health?

Of course, someone could equally argue that there are also religious faiths and leaders and places of worship in the world, but that none of these prove the existence of God. All that these things do is to provide evidence of organised religion. In one way, this argument by analogy is mistaken. (The argument is that the existence of places of worship doesn't prove the existence of God; so the existence of hospitals doesn't prove the existence of health.) It is a mistaken notion because in the case of 'health', there are what we might call 'observable phenomena', which hospitals and public health programmes and so on have clearly been set up to address. We walk into hospitals and see people who are sick and in need of what we easily call their 'health' being restored. Public health programmes have clearly been set up to counter a partic-ular problem; infectious diseases, smoking and so on. It seems easy for us to assert, at least in a superficial way, that success in reducing smoking, for example, is connected to 'health'. But we can't go into a place of worship, such as a church, and in a similar manner observe phenomena that would lead us to believe in the existence of God.

But in another way the analogy has a point. It's easily possible to imagine a religious person arguing that 'God' is present in places of worship such as churches. Of course, the non-religious person would probably dismiss this idea out of hand. There are, though, variations on that idea. Someone might suggest that 'God' isn't literally present in the church, but that the building (which might have been standing for hundreds of years) can be understood as an important symbol of God, or as a representation of a continued and powerful human belief in Him. Someone else might argue that God isn't just present in the church but is in fact everywhere. Yet another person could assert that when we talk of 'God', what in fact we are talking about is a strong human need to acknowledge and develop the spiritual aspect of our being. The point is that the empirical fact of systems and structures of organised religion might not lead us to believe that God (as in, for example, the God of the Old Testament) actually exists. But it would be hard to deny that they did not represent something very important about the nature of humanity; for example the spiritual aspect of ourselves, or the need we have to try and discover meaning beyond our everyday lives.

So thinking about this analogy in fact moves us forward, in this way:

▸ We can agree that organised religion doesn't prove the existence of God. It does, though, demonstrate the human search for Him.
▸ Organisations such as hospitals and practices such as medicine or nursing demonstrate the human search for health.
▸ The difficulty in both cases (God and 'health') is that we seem unable to agree on what constitutes the thing we seek. Is 'God' an active presence, or a component within us or a search for meaning? Is 'health' that which is produced by the work of hospitals and doctors and nurses, or is it far wider than just work trying to deal with disease and illness?

So we come to the idea that the central ontological questions for our field of study are about the *nature* of the existence of health, rather than whether it exists in the first place. What *actually* is it? What grounds are there for believing it to have the form and nature we consider it to have? And naturally following from these ontological questions are epistemological ones. If we think it has this or that particular form and nature, what then can we reasonably know about it? How can we know this? The relationship between the ontology and the epistemology of health is close and fundamental. Exploration of the nature of health requires us almost automatically to consider what and how we can know what we do about it, as the following contrasting examples demonstrate.

Health as the Absence of Disease: An Account from JG Scadding

Scadding, a physician and nosologist (nosology is the branch of medical science concerned with the classification of disease) argues that when we talk about 'disease', all we are doing is to apply convenient labels that relate to stages in the diagnostic process (Scadding, 1988).

The stages are:

▸ Clinical description (syndrome),
▸ disorder of structure (morbid anatomy),
▸ disorder of function (pathophysiology),
▸ causation (aetiology).

Imagine that a doctor sees a patient with a terrible cough. The doctor labels it chronic bronchitis. This is the clinical description she offers. She sends the patient for an X-ray, which identifies shadowed lungs (disorder of structure). A lung function test reveals severely limited lung capacity (disorder of function). Microbiological examination finally identifies tubercle bacilli in the patient's sputum. The aetiology of the cough and the patient's associated pain and discomfort (its causation) is tuberculosis.

'Disease' then, according to Scadding, is simply a description of abnormal phenomena present in living organisms. And if this is what 'disease' is, surely 'health' can be defined in a similarly tight way:

> If someone asks, 'Am I healthy?', all the doctor can do is to seek for evidences of known diseases and for significant deviations of structure and function from expected norms and reassure the enquirer if he finds none. (Scadding, 1988: 123)

So 'health' is no more and no less than the absence of abnormal structure and function. Health is quite simply the absence of disease. If we try to evaluate a person's 'health' in any other way than through the objective, demonstrable criteria of structural and functional normality or abnormality, we will be led only to muddle and confusion. We will open ourselves up to a range of unnecessary value judgements; meaningful description will become impossible.

Health as 'The Foundations for Achievement': An Account from David Seedhouse

Seedhouse's account and argument is quite different (Seedhouse, 1986, 2001). While Scaddding develops a tightly nominalist account of 'disease' and argues that 'health' can be accounted for in the same way, Seedhouse begins with the idea that 'health' is a contested concept. We can, though, locate a central theme in many existing accounts of health. This is the notion that 'work for health' is about removing obstacles to human potential, and these obstacles extend well beyond narrow biological and medical boundaries. So:

> Work for health is essentially *enabling*. It is a question of providing the appropriate foundations to enable the achievement of personal and group potentials. Health in its different degrees is created by removing obstacles and by providing the basic means by which biological and chosen goals can be achieved. . . . *A person's optimum state of health is equivalent to the set of conditions which enable a person to work to fulfil his or her realistic chosen and biological potentials. Some of these conditions are of the highest importance for all people. Others are variable dependent upon individual abilities and circumstances.* (Seedhouse, 1986: 61)

Reflecting on these separate accounts, their difference becomes clear. Scadding invests in a tightly nominalist account, one grounded, he believes, by objective evidence. After carefully examining someone, a doctor can turn round and say objectively, 'There is no structural abnormality. This person is therefore healthy.' Seedhouse's account, while equally rigorous in its argument, uses this to try and press home the idea that the 'evidence' for health depends to a large extent on interpretation. Beneath the overarching understanding that health is 'the foundations for achievement', it allows for a much wider range of explanations of 'health' in particular cases. For example, on Seedhouse's account, someone could be enduring significant degrees of 'structural abnormality' yet still be regarded as healthy. I know someone, for example, who suffers from a highly degenerative form of multiple sclerosis, yet continues to take pleasure in work and enjoys a wide range of positive friendships – things that allow the person to continue working towards achieving his human potential. It seems quite reasonable to suggest that despite his physical condition, this person is healthy. Equally, I have a friend who has no known physical ailment but for some time has been very dissatisfied with his life and circumstances. Would I want unambiguously to call him 'healthy'? I certainly might have difficulty in doing so and not just because a doctor might attribute a 'structural abnormality' (if that's what it can be called) such as depression to his state. The point of these two examples is to suggest that within certain broad limits, Seedhouse's account of health as 'the foundations for achievement' allows for quite a lot of interpretation about what health might actually consist of.

I don't want, for the moment, to engage in detailed examination and critique of these quite different accounts of the nature of health. This will be one of my tasks in Chapter 7. My intention right now is to connect these two separate ontological perspectives on 'health' to problems of epistemology. My key question at this stage is:

▸ What implications do the accounts have for issues to do with the nature of *knowledge about health* and how we can have that knowledge?

I want to argue that the two accounts lead to contrasting positions on health-related knowledge. These are the positions of the *objectivist* (emerging from Scadding's account) and the *interpretivist* (the position with which a Seedhouse – like view has more affinity).

Objectivism, Interpretivism and Health Knowledge

Scadding offers an objective account of health. Given what we know about the nature of disease, how can it possibly be meaningful to talk of health as anything other than disease absence? So our health-related knowledge must equally have objective dimensions. We must be able to point to objective, observable and indisputable facts in our talk about health. Seedhouse on the other hand, allows for interpretation to quite a large degree. Health is the foundations for achievement. It must surely be the case that such foundations are complex and unique to each individual. So our understanding of health must allow us (to some degree at least) to engage in interpretation as we try to work out what it might mean in particular contexts and for particular people.

Let's think first about the implications for epistemology of the objectivist position on health. If we believe that 'health' is an objective fact whose existence (or otherwise) can be subject to empirical observation, then we are making certain knowledge – related assumptions:

▸ There is an objective reality in the world whose nature we can understand.
▸ *Quantitative* methodology and the techniques and methods of quantitative investigation are best placed to help us identify and record the nature of this objective reality.
▸ We can undertake experiments, observe specific processes, gather statistics and measure so that the form, appearance and nature

of this reality become completely (and indisputably) clear to us (Holliday, 2002).

▸ We can develop hypotheses in relation to our areas of investigation and experiment to test these. In this way, our hypotheses can be proven or disproven.

Our enquiry, then, is a *positivist* one. That is to say, its limits are set by what can be firmly established through empirical observation and scientific method (Lacey, 1976). In the example of the patient with the terrible cough, say, scientific method leads to the doctor identifying tuberculosis. (The process of observation, hypothesis, testing and, experimentation leads to the diagnosis.)

But the health objectivist – positivist wouldn't want to confine explanations of the nature of health simply to the level of *individual* function or dysfunction. Through epidemiology, he or she would be concerned to map and understand the nature of disease (and so health) within and across populations (Mulhall, 2001), using techniques of measurement, hypothesis and testing on a much larger scale. The objectivist–positivist project of describing and explaining 'health' through quantitative enquiry is far reaching. It also shapes in a profound way social understanding of the nature of health, of knowledge about its nature and what can be done to maintain or improve it. Critical examination of this project will be a theme running through the whole of this book. For the moment, though, I simply want to argue that taking an objectivist ontological position on health leads to the adoption of positivism as the means of operating to find out more about its nature.

Let's move now to interpretivism. If I believe that what we understand by health is subject to interpretation, it follows that a quite different set of assumptions about the nature of our health-related knowledge, and what we need to do to extend it, will emerge:

▸ 'Reality' is not necessarily fixed. We all interpret it in different ways at different times. Some may even believe that 'reality' doesn't exist at all, but instead is constructed by individuals, through their experiences and circumstances (Holliday, 2002);

▸ So rather than engaging in pathological examination, we will be trying to explore how people feel, what motivates them, what kinds of attitudes they have, what beliefs they possess and how those beliefs are shaped (Poppay and Williams, 1994);

▸ Some of this exploration (possibly quite a large part) will involve a broadening of focus from just the person to the environmental and social circumstances in which that individual finds himself or herself;

‣ The focus will be on social and psychological processes, rather than on physical function (or functional abnormality);

‣ There will be a concern to elicit views from people, to observe their actions and reactions and interactions with others. So listening, talking and watching become the by-words of knowledge-seeking (Ball, 1990);

‣ Methods might include interviews, group discussions, structured or unstructured observation and so on;

‣ In these processes of listening, talking and watching the boundaries between the investigator and the investigated may become much less clear. For some, researcher engagement with the world being investigated might even become the method of research itself, as is the case with ethnography (Ball, 1990).

If these are the assumptions of the health interpretivist, the contrast with those of the objectivist seems marked. And if objectivist–positivists pursue their knowledge-seeking about health through quantitative methods, it might seem to follow that interpretivists will automatically align themselves with *qualitative* research paradigms and methods. But I'm reluctant to suggest this, at least in a blanket sense My argument now is that the nature of the health interpretivist's research style is rather more blurred than that of the objectivist. Simply aligning interpretivism with qualitative methodology is much more problematic than a relatively straightforward connection of the objectivist to positivism and quantitative methodology. If we recognise this, we start to expose difficulties with interpretivism, and with the place of qualitative research in health studies. We also begin to expose problems facing any project that seeks reasonable answers to the questions I began with: what can we know about health? How can we know it?

Biomedicine, Research and the Limits of Interpretivism

I start this argument about health research and the limits faced by interpretivism with a simple claim. It is that health interpretivists might choose on some occasions to use and rely on quantitative techniques. They might accept, for example, that the nature of 'health' depends on the meaning given it by individuals, groups or communities, but nevertheless still be interested in trying to discover if meaning is generalisable – say from one community to another. (The search for generalisability is of course a characteristic of quantitative research.) These are the motivations behind large-scale health and lifestyle surveys (e.g., Cox *et al.*, 1987; Cox *et al.*, 1993; Health Education Authority, 1995). Respondents to these kinds of surveys may be able to offer their own interpretations of 'health' and investigators will of course be interested in eliciting meaning. Nevertheless, results in the examples above are quantified. They are attempts at generalisability. The truth is that we can seek a broader understanding of the nature of health than a focused objectivist such as Scadding and in doing so may consider ourselves to be interpretivists. Nevertheless, we may still want to try and quantify our understanding.

Why is it more difficult to describe a firm alignment between interpretivism and qualitative methodology? I argue that there are three reasons. The first is that interpretivists, despite their search for personal meaning and broader, social explanation, are very often working in the profound shadow of biomedicine. Objective, biomedical understandings of 'disease' and 'health' are hugely influential in Western society (Turner, 2003). Biomedicine's belief (represented here by Scadding) that we can discover and deal with objective realities is extremely powerful and at the heart of a tradition that has dominated attitudes and practices related to the health domain at least since the Enlightenment of the eighteenth century (Tilford *et al.*, 2003). One result of this search for social understanding while working in the 'shadow of biomedicine' has been the development of a tradition of theorising and exploration of health and illness that can be seen as both complementary to, and supportive of, biomedical practices (Armstrong, 2003). This tradition has sought to use social science to explain health and disease in ways that emphasise the fundamental importance of biomedicine. Given this, it's understandable that the tradition has tried to work mainly in the same quantitative investigative paradigm as biomedicine itself. Doing so can be seen at least partly as a way of trying to demonstrate credibility to its powerful would-be benefactor.

The second reason is that it's possible to understand at least some (probably most) interpretivist positions as having limits. The interpretivist is not necessarily saying, 'Anything and everything is health, depending on what you think about health and what meaning you personally give to it.' Even quite a liberal interpretive position such as

'The Foundations for Achievement' has limits; we couldn't include anything that wasn't connected to the achievement of human potential. The problem of course is trying to work out what does in fact contribute to the achievement of human potential, and what doesn't. We could argue that certain things definitely do (a good education, say) and others definitely don't (enslavement is one thing that comes to mind). But there are a lot of things 'in the middle' that might or might not, depending on individual circumstances. (Smoking, driving a car and one-night stands are three such things that immediately occur to me. The point is not so much *what* limits have been set, *but the fact that limits have been set at all.*) Other interpretivist accounts of health are much more limiting than Seedhouse's. The argument developed by Downie, Tannahill and Tannahill, for example, is interpretive in the sense that the 'necessary personal and social values' (Downie, Tannahill and Tannahill, 1996: 158–161), which they argue must be present for individual and social flourishing (health) are presumably allowed to vary between groups, communities and societies. But any scope for interpretation is severely limited by the caveat that:

> There are. . . . better and worse lifestyles. . . . Unless we are convinced that some lifestyles are better than others. . . . we can see no point in health promotion. (Downie, Tannahill and Tannahill, 1996: 5)

In other words, Downie and colleagues are arguing that there are values we ought and others we ought not to accept as 'the values of health'. Their interpretivist position turns out to be highly limited.

Thinking Point

'There are better and worse lifestyles.' Is it possible to agree with this statement? Is it possible to *disagree?*

If interpretivist accounts of health have limits ('this can be health but this can't'), then our search for meaning will likewise be constrained. Placing constraints and limiting understanding make it more likely that a belief will develop that there is an unproblematic reality out there waiting to be discovered. This as I have said is the task of quantitative research.

The third reason for difficulty in ascribing a particular epistemological paradigm to interpretive positions on health is closely connected to the second, because it also concerns the accessibility of reality. I've just argued that circumscribed interpretivist positions make belief in a fixed, unproblematic reality more possible. This is an idea of reality inspired by views on the nature of health – that somehow what counts as 'health' needs to be curtailed. But the notion of a relatively limited, straightforward reality may also be inspired by beliefs connected to the nature of research and enquiry.

The health interpretivist may be attached to the project of understanding the meaning of health for individuals and communities through qualitative research. But between one researcher and another, there might be quite different ideas on what can be uncovered by such work and what it could mean. Within the broad span of qualitative research, it is possible to distinguish two distinctive paradigms; *naturalism*, and what Holliday (2002: 20) calls *progressivism*:

▸ *Naturalism* operates with the belief that reality is relatively straightforward, and that it can be captured by the researcher just so long as they immerse themselves in the research setting long enough and get to grips sufficiently with the accounts offered to them by those within the setting;

▸ *Progressivism* on the other hand, a term used to embrace a range of further paradigms including constructionism and post-modernism, believes that reality is not 'out there', waiting to be discovered. Instead the social world is constructed by people within it and researchers' interpretations of it (Hammersley and Atkinson, 1995).

So depending on the qualitative health researcher's position – whether naturalist or progressivist – she may be more or less inclined to believe in some kind of fixed reality, independent of herself and her own constructions. And if she is more inclined in this direction, once again the interpretivist may move to more of a determined position on the nature of health, one which might to some degree appear to resemble the positivism of the health objectivist.

In summary, the three arguments for the ambiguous commitment to the qualitative paradigm on the part of the health interpretivist are these:

▸ The interpretivist, like it or not, is working in the positivist 'shadow of biomedicine';

▸ Any reasonable interpretivist position places limits on what they understand by 'health'. In placing those limits, the interpretivist may come to believe that 'reality' is less problematic than perhaps it actually is;

▸ Depending on whether the interpretivist has an affinity towards naturalist or progressive qualitative research, once again their views on the nature of 'reality' and what needs to be done to uncover it will be circumscribed in some way.

Objectivism, Interpretivism and the Difficulty of Adopting a 'Middle Position' on the Nature of Health and Health Knowledge

This problem of connecting a particular investigative paradigm to health interpretivism seems to be a reflection of more general difficulties in thinking about the nature of health, what can be known about it and how we can know it. I began my discussion with two fairly representative accounts of separate positions on the nature of health itself: the objectivist (health is something that can be objectively defined); and the interpretivist (it has different meanings in different contexts, so making understanding and interpretation of meaning all-important). It's quite clear that an ontological tension exists between these two separate positions. There is little difficulty in imagining an objectivist and an interpretivist meeting and being completely unable to agree on the nature of existence of the thing, whatever it is, that they both choose to call 'health'.

But it is conversely very hard to believe that the two will 'agree to differ'. As I've argued, separate decisions about the nature of health lead to different ways of trying to understand and investigate its nature. In broad terms, the objectivist, believing it is possible objectively to describe and classify 'health', will gravitate towards the positivist paradigm and choose to work with quantitative methodologies. After all, if someone believes that 'health' can be observed and described, it makes sense also to believe that it can be measured, that it's possible to engage in scientific tests to establish greater knowledge about its nature, and so on. On the other hand, the interpretivist holds the belief that much depends on subjective meaning when we think about the idea of 'health'. So they might naturally incline towards qualitative methodologies to explore the nature of that meaning for individuals and communities and the contextual influences that play a part in shaping meaning. Then again, as I've argued, one way or another limits to interpretivism may have been established and an inclination to quantitative enquiry on the part of the interpretivist might have been set. The potential for dispute extends, then, into epistemology, compounding the ontological disagreement with which we began. Moreover, the dispute isn't simply one of objectivist versus interpretivist. It also involves interpretivists in dispute with each other, too (the naturalist against the progressivist, for example).

Perhaps there seems to be an obvious, common sense answer to all of this. Why can't we just accept that the idea of 'health' contains both objective elements ('Surely it must in some way be about the absence of disease!') and interpretive or subjective ones ('There's no reason why my idea of health shouldn't differ from yours?)' This seems like a perfectly reasonable response. To some extent, it is the lesson that can be drawn from considering so-called lay accounts of health that have emerged in recent years. As I will argue, though, there is difficulty in reconciling complex lay accounts of health with the polarised theoretical positions we have so far considered.

Lay Accounts of Health

Lay accounts are those which emerge from empirical research of some kind; research which aims to elicit the understanding of 'ordinary' people on the idea of 'health'. Such work has also encountered perspectives on the related concepts we have been discussing – for example, 'disease' (Lupton, 1994). Emerging as they do from a complex world, lay accounts of health seem to expose the falsity within the dichotomous objectivist versus interpretivist debate that we have been considering; a debate that only serves to emphasise the difficulties in getting an adequate purchase on the idea of 'health'.

Accounts of health from ordinary people demonstrate two important things:

▸ The importance of culture and who we are within cultures (e.g. our age, gender and so on) in shaping understandings of the nature of health;
▸ The struggle to extend talk about health beyond the confines imposed by medicine ('health as disease absence'), while also to some degree subsuming to the power of medical discourse and practice and incorporating it within accounts.

Although this brief review of lay accounts that follows focuses on those that have been developed in relatively recent times, it is important to be reminded that accounts of health can be traced back through history (Downie and Macnaughton, 2001). One important lesson of a historically more lengthy examination of accounts of health is that it would serve to demonstrate the relative dominance, within present day stories, of the medical 'body as a machine' view of health and disease. In this sense, contemporary lay accounts represent the struggle between holism and reductionism in ideas about health that, as I've briefly discussed, stems from the eighteenth century Enlightenment and its project of rational understanding of our world and ourselves. This struggle, and its major implications for understanding health and its study forms a theme of this book as a whole and will be discussed especially in Chapter 9.

Various studies have emphasised the importance of culture and more particularly who we are within a given culture in determining how we view health. (See, for example, Herzlich, 1973; Williams, 1983; Cox *et al.*, 1987.) Such things as age, class and gender all play important roles in establishing how we account for health. Cox and colleagues, for example, pointed to the general emphasis within younger people on the importance of 'physical fitness' as an aspect of health, whereas respondents overall to their study (with an age range of 18–60+) emphasised '*psychological* fitness' in their accounts. This is representative of a tendency within lay accounts of health to become more complex and multilayered according to the greater age of the respondent (Hardey, 1998). Secondary analyses of Cox *et al*'s data also revealed distinctions of cultural identity. For example, respondents from Afro-Caribbean backgrounds placed importance on physical fitness within their accounts, whereas those from Asian backgrounds drew out more the idea of health as a capacity to function (Howlett *et al.*, 1991; Ahmad, 1993). Social class plays an important part, too, in framing conceptions. For example, Calnan and Johnson (1985), analysing responses from both working-class and middle-class women living in London, found differences in how the separate respondents viewed factors contributing to health. The middle-class women, in talking about 'health', referred to things like being active and eating the right food; whereas the working-class women talked about it as the thing that 'helped them get through the day'.

The struggle to move talk of health beyond the confines of simply 'the absence of disease' is evident in many lay accounts of health. While the middle class respondents from Paris and Normandy in Herzlich's classic account of health beliefs (Herzlich, 1973) talked of the idea of health as disease absence ('health in a vacuum'), they also spoke of it as a 'reserve of strength' and 'equilibrium', an awareness of self and body. Equally, Williams (1983), in his analysis of the beliefs of the group of elderly people from Aberdeen with whom he worked, was moved towards the view that health for these people embraced more holistic notions. He writes:

> Hence although health can be used simply to mean the absence of disease, it is also used in a far more complex and positive sense; and this positive sense often dominated discussion by my samples of the relation of health to activity and moral effort. (Williams, 1983: 189)

And in their study of mothers in South Wales whose husbands were skilled manual workers, Pill and Stott (1982) found that some of these (interestingly, those with higher levels of formal education) described 'health' as something that was engendered by a positive and dynamic relationship between individuals and their environment.

This draws us towards a further theme in lay accounts of health; the degrees to which people believe they have control over their own health. Despite the rise of medicine and its frequent portrayal as technologically infallible in its ability to counter disease (and so produce 'health'), many lay accounts regard the ability to stay healthy as a matter of luck, and the forces of disease and illness as capricious in who they attack. This is especially so in accounts from working class respondents (Blaxter and Paterson, 1982; Cornwell, 1984). On the other hand, some lay accounts of health emphasise the capacity of individuals (if they have clear senses of power and purpose) to move towards 'health' in the much wider sense of achievement of life goals. These kinds of less fatalistic accounts of vulnerability to health and disease tend to emerge from middle class respondents (McGuire, 1988).

This brief review of lay accounts of health gives an impression of their depth and richness. In the light of such accounts, it seems possible to suggest the following:

▸ Lay accounts, in their complexity and variety, seem to suggest that ideas about health emerge from our cultural experience and location (age, gender, social circumstance, and so on);

▸ To this extent, the accounts are *constructions* by people trying to make sense of a world that is difficult to understand, and of their experience within it, rather than *descriptions* of any sort of objective reality;

▸ To talk of health in the theoretical terms of either the objectivist or the interpretivist simply isn't enough. Lay accounts move between and beyond these positions, relating 'health' to a variety of sources and states, some within and some beyond the control of individuals.

Back to the Difficulty of the 'Middle Position' for the Health Studies Student

If lay accounts of health with all their richness and complexity can both recognise the sense of seeing health partly as 'the absence of disease' but also have the wisdom to recognise that it must also in some ways extend beyond this, why is this difficult for theorists of health? And why in turn, given their involvement with health theorists, is it difficult for health studies students?

Part of the problem lies in the very complexity of lay accounts. Their shades and nuances do not correspond easily with the strident claims of theorists seeking to control or eliminate ambiguity. As I've claimed, the positivist outlook of biomedicine towers over dispute. A natural result of this is to set limits to any interpretivist position on health (for example Downie *et al.*'s 'better and worse lifestyles') and so in some way (even if only broadly) gravitate towards a more objectivist standpoint. Gravitational force is increased by the naturalist position on research – attractive to at least some interpretivists – with its belief that there is indeed a reality ('the reality of health') waiting to be discovered somewhere, if only we can look long and hard enough. All this often militates against careful consideration of the rich and involved perspectives of lay people (Lupton, 1994).

So the possibility of a reasonable 'middle position' on the nature of health and health knowledge is clouded for theorists and students by the broad dominance of positivism in the field of health studies. But the reasonable position for us as learners and teachers is clouded not only by the ontological and epistemological debates I have discussed in this chapter. It is also substantially blurred by what lies behind the positions we might take up in relation to these debates. Our positions, I argue, are very often based not on rational consideration of whatever evidence might exist for them, but rather on *ideologies*. These ideologies are themselves framed by our personal, occupational and professional experiences and beliefs – *including, fundamentally, our experiences and beliefs as learners and teachers*. This is the next stage of my argument for the difficulty of health studies, and the main focus of Chapter 2.

Turning Point?

Turning Points appear at the end of most chapters in this book. Their purpose is to encourage you to think again, and perhaps think differently, about some or all of the material contained in the chapter and the arguments that I have presented or developed.

This turning point relates to the idea of health as a contested concept. A great deal rests on this idea. If we accept the notion, it is relatively easy to go down the interpretivist road. If we are doubtful about it, the objectivist position beckons. An important premise for David Seedhouse's argument that health is 'the foundations for achievement' relates to the idea of health as a contested concept. His argument takes into account and to some extent draws on the work of the philosopher of history, WB Gallie. Initially Gallie (1956) identifies five necessary conditions, which must be fulfilled if a concept is to be regarded as what he calls 'essentially contested'. The conditions are:

1. The concept must be *appraisive* (i.e., it signifies a valued achievement);
2. While worth is attributed to the achievement as a whole, there must be an internal complexity to and within it;
3. Thus we must be able to argue about what, for us, are the most important features of the concept (and different people will prioritise features differently);
4. The achievement signified by the concept must be modifiable in the light of changing circumstances;
5. Use of an essentially contested concept means to use it 'both aggressively and defensively' (Gallie, 1956: 172).

He later identifies two further conditions, claiming that the first five are necessary, but not sufficient. A concept could fulfil conditions 1–5 but still not be 'essentially contested' – rather it could simply be 'radically confused'. The two further conditions are:

6. There must be, historically, an original exemplar of the concept, acknowledged by all who contest it;

7. Current 'competition' on the use of the concept must enable the original exemplar's achievement to be sustained and developed (Gallie, 1956: 180).

Seedhouse (1986) is doubtful of the idea of a 'true historical exemplar' for health and so seems to reject conditions 6 and 7 in relation to the concept of health. But he does argue that it must be possible to discover a 'contemporary uncontested general sense of health' (Seedhouse, 1986: 25). Which of these seven conditions do you think applies to the concept of health? Is Seedhouse right to argue on the one hand for 'no historical exemplar', but on the other for his 'contemporary uncontested general sense'? Does holding both these separate positions square up? If his claim for the 'general sense' doesn't emerge from history, where does it come from?

While we might instinctively feel greater sympathy for a more relative, interpretivist position such as Seedhouse's, it's also possible to argue that the current dominant 'uncontested general sense' of health is the notion of it being 'absence of disease' – in other words, the objectivist position. Moreover, we could further argue that one strong contestant for the 'original, historical exemplar' of health is in fact health as disease absence. Thus an alternative way of constructing arguments about the nature of health is to suggest that we are talking about an essentially contested concept, and that our arguing derives from the historical exemplar of health as the absence of disease.

If this is the case, then *both* the health interpretivists and the health objectivists have got it wrong. The interpretivists are wrong because they are failing to allow the essential importance of the original exemplar. And the objectivists are wrong because they are failing to allow the importance of dispute which, if Gallie is right, actually serves to strengthen the exemplar.

In the light of this brief discussion of health as (potentially at least) an 'essentially contested concept' – in Gallie's terms – review the arguments of the objectivist and the interpretivist that have been considered in this chapter. Does it make any difference to your initial reactions and your own position?

What's gone on in this chapter?

I've described and discussed two broad ontological positions on the nature of health – objectivism and interpretivism. The separate epistemological implications of these different positions have been considered. Both harbour problems for the health studies student. It seems odd to think of 'health' as simply the absence of disease, but if we try and engage in more interpretive positions, it appears as if we often have limits set – or we set limits for ourselves – on what these interpretations might involve. My next step is to connect these limits to our own experiences of 'health' – particularly our occupational, professional and learning and teaching experiences.

2 Professional Identity and the Study of Health

What is this chapter going to do?

My next step in this argument for the complexity of health studies is to connect the limits that seem to be placed on our understanding of health to our own experiences – particularly our occupational, professional and learning and teaching experiences. I argue in this chapter that the nature of the health care professions and our experiences of being health care professionals guide us towards certain ways of understanding what 'health' is. Broadly, becoming and being a professional points us in the direction of objectivist understandings of the concept – 'health as the absence of disease'. This poses problems in terms of our capacity to think about health in new or alternative ways.

Professional Order and Professional Identity

The possibility of adopting 'reasonable' positions on the nature of health and its study is obscured, I've argued, by the deep-seated ontological and epistemological disputes discussed in Chapter 1. Now the problem becomes deeper still. My argument is that as professionals, we are encouraged – possibly even obliged – to accept one or other of the ontological and epistemological positions I have already described. Our profession, and our own professional identity and background shape to a significant extent our views on the nature of health. These mould our ideas on what we can know about health and what we think we ought to be doing to improve it (Armstrong, 1983; Eraut, 1994). Moreover, as a result of being the professionals that we are, we promulgate, strengthen and reinforce these views so that they are embedded further still within our profession, whatever it happens to be. I don't want to deny that professions can be challenged. But I do want to suggest that doing so is likely to be very difficult.

Professional Identity: The Theory

What does it mean to be a professional? There are at least two ways of understanding the nature of professional identity:

▸ We can *describe* what somebody has to *do* and how they have to *behave* in order to be regarded as 'a professional'.
▸ We can think particularly about what they have to *believe* and how they have to believe it in order to develop and maintain their status as 'a professional' (Hoyle, 1980; Eraut, 1994).

Thinking Point

What does the idea of being a 'professional' mean to you?

If we think about describing the development, action and behaviour of the professional, we would probably come up with the following things:

▸ Involvement in a relatively long period of specialist training in order to become a member of the profession concerned;
▸ The need to be admitted to a carefully regulated register of the profession's practitioners once that training has been successfully completed;
▸ The need to keep to the profession's code of conduct, which prescribed and guided the professional's actions and behaviour towards patients or clients;
▸ The requirement to support (even if only tacitly) the profession's efforts to develop knowledge about how it could be more effective and serve its public better (Hoyle, 1980; Eraut, 1994).

But in developing a descriptive account of what it is to be a professional we not only have to consider what professionals do and how they behave, but also what *beliefs* underpin their action and behaviour. Indeed, becoming a professional, in the sense of learning what to do and how to act, are processes that are fed by parallel and reciprocal ones in which the professional in training learns what beliefs they should possess and what values ought to be important to them. So:

▸ Professionals learn what to do and how to do it.

But they also:

▸ Learn what to believe and what to value.

Importantly, these are not beliefs and values that professionals in training can select or reject in a 'pick-n-mix' sort of way. Nor are they values that they develop for themselves, through their own free-thinking. They are the beliefs and values *of the profession itself*. And part of belonging to that profession involves assuming these beliefs and values. These beliefs and values might include, for example:

▸ The *belief* that the profession performs a crucial social function. So there is essential *value* in its work;
▸ The *belief* that the exercise of this function requires considerable skill. So this skill is itself a *value* and to be encouraged through both initial education and training, and continuing professional development;
▸ The *belief* that this skill should be exercised for the benefit of patients and clients. So the *values* of concern and respect for these people become central;
▸ The *belief* that because the profession's skill is so specialised, it should be allowed freedom to determine how it practices. So the *value* of professional autonomy also becomes key (Hoyle, 1980: 45).

Thinking Point

Does this account of the beliefs and values inherent within the idea of 'the profession' correspond with your own views about how your profession (if you belong to one) sees itself? If not, where does the difference lie?

The net result of these parallel and reciprocal processes of learning what to do on the one hand, and learning what to believe and value on the other, is that professional action and professional values become very closely enmeshed. It's hard to imagine it otherwise. Take, for example, the profession of nursing – and a relatively straightforward nursing action such as washing a patient. At one level, this simply involves the activity of washing someone. At another, though, there is a skill and expertise involved (e.g., assessing and taking care of pressure areas, or observing for visible signs of infection). At yet another level, all of this is being done in a way that we could characterise as 'caring' and entailing respect for the patient being cared for. It is difficult to understand this as an activity of professional nursing unless all these components – the action, its implicit skill, the values underlying it – are present.

Perhaps as importantly, there is a strong sense in which *all of us* (whether nurses or not) are aware of the values underpinning this example of nursing action, and nursing in general. We have this awareness because we recognise the importance of the profession of nursing and the crucial function it performs in our 'society of strangers' (Larson, 1977).

Our society is one whose size and complexity means that we have to decide collectively, and not individually, who provides us with goods such as 'caring'. We have decided that nursing is one of the professions providing us with this good and so we have a natural interest in the beliefs and values of nursing (Koehn, 1994). This is one of the reasons why we are all so shocked when those values are disrupted, as in the case of Beverley Allitt, the child-murdering paediatric nurse who in her actions appeared to represent the antithesis of nursing values (Hart, 2004).

Of course it's still possible, despite this very powerful collective sense of the values of nursing, to dispute or reject these values. This is possible simply because of the nature of values themselves. At the most basic level, we can understand values as those things that we find valuable. By itself, though, this is hardly a helpful understanding, as with even the most cursory thought, we probably realise that we regard many different things as valuable. I personally value, for example, ice cream and chocolate, books and music, family and the freedom to follow my career and my interests. But recognising in this way that we hold multiple values leads also to realisation that not all of our values are of the same kind. I value ice cream and chocolate, but not in the same way as I value even novels and music, or certainly family and freedom. The value I place on ice cream and chocolate is to do with my liking them. So I could call them 'liking' or *subjective* values (Dworkin, 1995). I like books and music, too, but I value them especially because they help me to relax, to leave the everyday world for a while and imagine other possibilities. So they provide me with things that I want or need (relaxation, escape) and thus have *instrumental* value (Dworkin, 1995). Family and freedom are different kinds of values again, because while they are things that I both like and find useful, I cannot reduce them entirely to preference or utility. I like my family, say, and need them in the sense of the emotional succour they provide to me – but I cannot see them wholly in these terms. Their value extends beyond use or liking. It wouldn't be odd to talk about freedom, say, as something that characterised (or ought to characterise) what it is to be human itself. So when we hear of people being deprived of their freedom for no reason, or for reasons that we can't agree with, we may well regard those who are taking it away as removing an essential component of being human, and so in our eyes they become *inhuman* themselves. (Think, for example, of the Nazis and their removal of Jewish people, among others, to concentration camps.) That these kinds of values play a central part in determining what it is to be human make them fundamental or *intrinsic* values (Dworkin, 1995).

So, we can consider there are values that are:

‣ *Subjective* (I just happen to like X, so I value it);
‣ *Instrumental* (X is useful to me, so I value it);
‣ *Intrinsic* (X is so fundamental to being human that because I am human, I have to value it).

Thinking Point

Consider some of the things that are valuable in your own life. Which of these might be regarded as *subjective*? As *instrumental*? As *intrinsic*?

We can certainly imagine dispute occurring in relation to subjective and instrumental values. ('Of course plain chocolate is better than milk chocolate!'; 'I can't understand why you think classical music is better than jazz!') But dispute is also possible in relation to intrinsic values, and it is dispute of a particularly difficult sort. Although I might believe that freedom, for example, is an intrinsic value, someone else may not share my belief. While it's hard to know quite where to begin in arguing with someone who rejects the importance of human freedom completely (how come they reject it but nevertheless feel free enough to argue with me?) it's a little easier to imagine someone with a different *conception* of freedom to mine. It is maybe easier still to think of somebody who holds different views to mine about, say, the relative importance of individual freedom. They may believe, for example, that on occasions someone's personal freedom is worth sacrificing for more collective communitarian concerns. Perhaps this is the motivation underpinning acts of revolt and revolution, or of national defence. Antony Beevor, for example, writes of the Russian state of mind as millions prepared to defend their country against German attack in the Second World War.

> The recruiting poster, 'The Motherland Calls!', showed a typical Russian woman holding the military oath and backed by a sheaf of bayonets . . . . Huge sacrifices were expected. 'Our aim is to defend something greater than millions of lives,' wrote a young tank commander in his diary exactly a month after the [German] invasion. "I am not speaking about my own life. The only thing to be done is to lose it to some advantage for the Motherland". (Beevor, 1999: 27–28)

Some people would find this idea of collective sacrifice for a greater ideal easily understandable. For others, it might appear bemusing. But the point of this dramatic example is to emphasise that our own positions on the nature of intrinsic values can differ from those of others, and separate positions are likely to be fundamentally fixed and entrenched. From this, I want to suggest that dispute about intrinsic values is likely to be especially acrimonious, protracted and perhaps even irresolvable.

My argument now is that the set of values we possess as a result of being a particular kind of professional (a nurse, say) can best be understood as at least in part a set of *intrinsic* values. They can't be completely understood as only subjective or only instrumental. Consider the set of possible 'professional nursing values' I described above – the value of the skills of nursing, respect for patients and clients and so on. There are, of course, probably ways of understanding this sort of set of values as subjective. ('I enjoy using my nursing skill.') We might also be able to understand them as instrumental. ('Respecting patients and clients is one way of ensuring that we do our job more efficiently because if we do so they are more likely to co-operate with us.') But they can't *only* be instrumental or subjective. If I was a member of the profession of nursing, holding the set of values I've described, I'd probably be quite worried by someone who thought that holding the value of patient respect was *all* to do with getting the job done with greater efficiency. I'd want to assert, probably quite strongly, that the value was at least partly intrinsic. There is a need to hold the value of respect for patients because patients *just do deserve our respect.*

But of course if professional values can be understood at least partly as intrinsic values, then they are lain open to the same kind of acrimonious and possibly irresolvable dispute as any other intrinsic value. I might agree with some or all of the values, or I might not. I might choose not to challenge them. Equally I might.

Let's continue with the nursing example for a little longer. A list of possible nursing values (the worth of nursing skill, respect for patients etc.) can be understood and interpreted in two different ways:

▸ We can understand the values *positively*. They are part of the basic foundations of the profession of nursing. This profession meets an essential societal need that would otherwise be lacking and so the values possess intrinsic importance.

▸ But we might understand them *negatively*. We might argue that while society does have an essential need for nursing skills, there is no reason why it should be the *profession of nursing* that supplies these. The value of professional nursing skill could be regarded as limiting or even disregarding of lay experiences and contributions to the processes of caring: the value of professional autonomy might be seen as simply a licence for the profession to do what it wants; and so on. Consequently the set of intrinsic values fundamental to the profession is disputed.

Critiques of professions, their purpose and values on these lines are strong elements within the discourses of some of the academic disciplines contributing to an understanding of health and health studies, such as sociology and philosophy. (See, for example, Halmos, 1971; Illich, 1975, 1977; Zola, 1972). In fact, one of the themes in Part III of this book is the potential for tension between academic critique of health care professionals and what they do; and the desire for support and direction from academics that those professionals understandably have.

So agreement or disagreement on a particular set of professional values (say, those of nursing) will be deep-seated and possibly irresolvable. Because our views are expressions of values, it may be extremely hard for us to engage in reasoned analysis of alternative positions. It may well be problematic also for others to engage in reasoned analysis of our own position. The nature of professional identity and professional values provides a ground for long-running and bitter disputes.

What Has all this Got to do with Health Studies?

This is a reasonable question. All you've done, you might say, is to suggest that professions exert a strong influence on our values. You've done no more than claim that our own professional identity is formed not simply by what we do (our actions), but also by what we believe (our values), and that the two are intertwined in complex ways with each other. How does this relate to your so-called difficulty of health studies?

The answer to the question is this. Part of our professional identity as a health care professional comprises of a set of beliefs about the nature of health, and the kind of value that health is. My claim now is that our professions naturally incline towards particular – perhaps generally positivist – conceptions of 'health' (Blaxter, 1990; Katz and Peberdy, 2001; Seedhouse, 1986, 2001). These conceptions in turn sharply inform the range of professional values that shape our practice, the kinds of things I have been talking about in this chapter (professional function, skills and so on). Because there is such a complex relationship between what we *do* as professionals and what we *believe*, our daily actions in the field of health will reinforce the values underpinning them. If my values orient broadly towards understanding the value of health as one of 'disease absence', I will regard the value of professional function as in some way to be involved with dealing with illness or disease. I will understand the value of its skills as being largely concerned about the treatment of illness or disease, and so on.

The net result of all this – values reinforcing actions and vice versa – is that 'positions' on health become fixed. It gets hard to engage in reasoned analysis of alternative views. The nature of the value of health is for me, say, 'the absence of disease'. My view of the value will then be fundamentally connected to other, complementary, values and principles, which together are mutually reinforcing and form my *ideology* of health, where ideology is understood as:

> A systematic set of principles linking perceptions of the world to explicit moral values . . . . [claimed by those promoting it as] better than any alternative. (Andrain and Apter, 1995: 4–25)

So here is the nub of the difficulty of professional identity and health studies: *Our professional identity makes it hard to view and understand the concept of health (along with related concepts and practices) in new or different ways.*

Clarifying the difficulty in this way assumes that, you think that it is actually important to try and examine new and different ways of thinking about and examining health. This isn't an unreasonable assumption; it would be hard to imagine why otherwise you might be engaged in the study of health. Even if our starting point for study involves thinking that our existing position on the nature of health is the one that in fact we want to stick to, we need to move away from it and examine others before we return to the place from which we started out. If we fail to do so, our perspectives will be neither critical nor reflective. My claim is that whether we believe we need to change how we think, or whether we need to confirm that what we think is right for us, our professional identities may well stand in the way.

This is not to deny that it can't be done. Both things are possible. David Armstrong, for example, in his book 'Political Anatomy of the Body' (1983), describes his experience as a medical student. Inculcated as he sees it through his professional training into a position where he saw health and illness as objective realities, his reading took him to Michel Foucault and the challenge offered by the French philosopher to such notions. Much of Armstrong's professional career since then has been about exposing what he regards as the myths of 'the stable body' and 'the objective reality' of disease (and health). These myths, in his view, have been used by medicine as a kind of 'power base' over the last two centuries. From this base, the profession has extended its control so that now we are all willing and active participants in the medicalisation of every aspect of our lives and social relationships (Armstrong, 1993). I will be discussing some of Armstrong's ideas in more detail in Chapter 9. The point I want to make now is that Armstrong offers an example of changing position on the nature of disease (and health) despite pressing professional identities and imperatives.

But while reviewing or altering your position on the nature of health is certainly not impossible, it is also not easy. And if the theoretical argument I've constructed about the power of professional identity and its impact on capacity for critical perspectives on health has not yet convinced you, perhaps the next step is to consider personal experience.

Professional Identity: The Experience

I began my own 'career in health' at the end of 1981, when I started training to become a Registered General Nurse (RGN). At the time,

I had no conception that I was embarking on a 'career in health'. In fact, it would probably have sounded odd to me if somebody had described it in that way. 'A career in health care', or 'a career in the Health Service' might possibly have sounded less strange, although of course neither of these things would have been likely to involve thinking about 'health' in the way that I am trying to do so in this book. 'Health care' and 'the health service' would have been understood as being largely about dealing with the 'objective reality of disease' (as indeed it's quite possible to argue that they still are today). The techniques for dealing with this objective reality were performed mainly in hospital, a place according to Armstrong that was 'ushered in' from the end of the nineteenth century onwards as this reality was discovered and efforts were begun to deal with it:

> The hospital [was] a place in which bodies could be examined with proper rigour, the post-mortem [was] the event in which the true nature of disease was finally revealed, and the many facets of clinical method which still underpin medical practice today [were engaged in]. (Armstrong, 1993: 55)

So I started my 'career in nursing' (which I suppose is what it should have been most properly called) in a hospital, learning mainly about the 'objective reality' of disease and the place of nursing in dealing with this. To begin with (in fact for quite a long time) there was hardly any doubt in my mind that I was actually engaged in training that was about developing the professional skills required to deal with disease as an objective reality – and its equally objective opposite state of 'health'. I was, I suppose, operating with an understanding of health that was closely akin to that of JG Scadding, referred to in Chapter 1, although my reasoning could hardly have been said to have been as explicit as that. The theoretical learning that I undertook in the first few weeks of training mainly centred around anatomy and physiology, the structure and function of bodies and their component parts, how they worked when healthy, what went wrong when they became diseased, and the effects resulting from dysfunction. In important ways, beginning a 'career in health' like this makes sense. As SH Cedar and Judy Hubbard express it:

> For most people, health is associated first and foremost with a physical state of being. Having a knowledge of physiological frameworks, pathways and mechanisms contributes to our understanding of this physical state of being. (Cedar with Hubbard, 2001: 37)

And of course this kind of common sense representation of the importance of physiology and bio-mechanical understanding of health and disease reflects the cultural dominance of science (including bio-medicine) in our field of interest. We need to know how to deal with disease (and so create health) because these things are largely understood in scientific and biomedical ways:

> With the process of modernisation, health and illness. . . . eventually became embraced by various scientific discourses. In Western medicine, disease entities became increasingly differentiated and disease states more specified as the human body is itself differentiated into its component parts. (Turner, 2003: 10)

This theoretical learning that I undertook, with its focus on the apparent objective realities of 'disease' and 'health', was a precursor to going out as a student nurse, along with others who were beginning their training, onto the wards. 'On the job' we learned, or tried to learn, the central skills involved in nursing, of caring for those whose physical states were disrupted, who were in some way 'dis-eased' and needed to be returned to 'health'. But as I engaged in this skills learning, I was also involved in another process – a process that generally was less overt than the explicit 'learning what to do' one. This was the process of *learning and beginning to assume the values and beliefs of nursing*.

The theoretical distinction I've already drawn between 'learning what to do' and 'learning what to believe' was firmly borne out through my practical experience while I was training to be a nurse. Along with learning how to take pulses and temperatures and blood pressures, how to dress wounds and deal with pressure sores, how to make beds and wash immobile patients, I learned what I should believe and what values I ought to hold. I learned that I was a beginning apprentice, at the lowest point of an enormous hierarchy. I learned that with persistence, and with respect for others further up this hierarchy (e.g., sisters on the wards where I was allocated), I could advance through it myself. I learned about the nature of the relationship between nurses and medical practitioners, that there were limits to the nursing role, but that there was co-dependency between nurses and doctors and that in some fairly indefinable way nurses had quite a large degree of control in the hospital system. (One way or another, sisters always seemed to be the ones who were *actually* in charge of wards!) I was learning all these things in high-pressure environments – acute medical and surgical wards, accident and emergency departments and intensive care units. This was also being learnt while I was working in ways that physically I'm certain I couldn't manage any more. I was standing up for most of an eight-hour shift, having (if I was lucky) maybe two half-hour breaks within this time. I was probably walking the equivalent of 20 miles a day as I rushed up and down the ward, between different beds and patients. I was finishing on a Late at 10 in the evening and having to be up at six the following morning to be in time for an Early. Not to mention the mind and body-numbing phenomenon of night shifts!

The net result of all this was that my life became synonymous with nursing. I came to share the set of nursing beliefs and values, such as the occupation having a crucial social function and its entitlement to be allowed to get on with performing this. Most importantly for the argument I am making here, I believed that the value of nursing lay in its caring for patients so that they recovered from disease and illness. So for me as a nurse in training all those years ago, 'health' *simply was* the absence of disease, the thing that you restored to (physically) sick people. The events and processes I've described profoundly influenced my view of the nature and value of health. This view emerged from my own difficult, heady, exhilarating and frightening socialisation into professional values (Hoyle, 1980). Crucially, the values that I was being required to accept (because this was what was happening) were never necessarily made explicit. Yet somehow, through the length and intensity and all-embracing nature of my experiences, I just did become aware (consciously or subconsciously) of what they were.

Professional Identity and the Difficulty of Health Studies

Joining theory of professional identity together with my own experiences leads us to the nub of the problem. Learning what to do and learning what to believe come together in the experience of 'professional socialisation' and an important element of this socialisation is our orientation towards a particular sort of conception of the value of health. Our view of the value tends towards the objective, health as 'the absence of disease' – closer to Scadding perhaps than to Seedhouse.

There are at least two possible arguments against my conception of the problem of professional identity and health studies:

▸ What I have just described is my own experience and cannot possibly be said to represent anything other than that;

▶ Even if what I've described as happening all those years ago did mean anything to anyone beyond myself, things have changed since then! Recent reforms of health care professional education and training curricula have completely altered the way professionals think about disease, and about health. Patients are no longer machines with broken bits that need to be fixed. We are all encouraged (obliged, perhaps) to see them in much more holistic ways, to take a fundamental interest in their broader lives and social circumstances. (See, for example, English National Board for Nursing, Midwifery and Health Visiting, 1987; General Medical Council, 1993.) Given this, how is it possible to persist with the idea that professionals hold very narrow views of the value of health?

These are potentially convincing arguments. Certainly I'm happy to admit to the accusation that my experience wasn't representative. This was, of course, what happened to me at that particular time. I don't have very much idea of whether it is an experience that others have shared. However, it is worth considering whether it resonates with your own.

Thinking Point

> If you've gone through a period of professional training, to what extent does my account of my own intensely involving experience match with your own memories of induction into your particular profession? What impact do you think your experience has had on your present understandings of the idea of 'health' and its nature as a value?

There is a need also to think about the experience of thinkers and writers who have at one time or another been practitioners and have recounted their perceptions of professional influences on conceptions of health-writers such as Armstrong, as well as others like Sam Porter (Porter, 1995). The impression from reading writers such as these is of their struggle to overcome the dominance of the 'medical model' of the human body as a machine with broken bits that need to be fixed. It's also worth reminding ourselves of the literature (often based on empirical work) that suggests the dominance of narrow, 'absence of disease' conceptions of health in professional thinking (Blaxter, 1990; Katz and Peberdy, 2001; Seedhouse, 2001).

But if there have been far-reaching policy and curricula changes that have encouraged us to think in broader ways about our patients or clients and their health, why do relatively narrow conceptions continue to dominate thinking? One answer to this question lies in the extent of what we might call 'medical imperialism'. Medicine and the so-called medical model are just so dominant that it is very hard to escape their influence, despite the best efforts of educational reform.

A more interesting and complex answer to the question lies in understanding of the process of socialisation into professional values itself. As I have said, the process is very often an implicit and subliminal one. To this extent, it has an important relationship with the idea of the 'hidden' or 'implicit' curriculum (Eisner, 1985; Cribb and Bignold, 1999). This is the idea that there is a set of unwritten professional rules that govern development and behaviour much more profoundly than the formal written curriculum itself. Students have to follow these unwritten rules if they want to 'get on' and become accepted as a member of the profession concerned.

The relationship between the 'hidden' curriculum and the process of socialisation into professional values is a close and reciprocal one. We learn the nature of what is 'hidden' and act in ways that express our acceptance of these tacit rules. In doing so, we conform to the expectations of the profession and demonstrate our commitment to its values. And in turn the process of socialisation comes, at least partly, to represent our commitment to following such essential hidden rules.

My contention is that the 'hidden' curriculum for many health care professionals in training involves unwritten rules and assumptions about the nature of the value of health. Whether or not you agree with this contention, a further example from my own experience might help stimulate thought on this idea.

Towards the end of my professional training in nursing, the idea of the Nursing Process assumed significance, at least in educational terms. The Nursing Process advocates seeing the patient as a whole person, in their social context, with a range of health needs – not just physical needs but also emotional, social and psychological ones (Roper, 1976). The idea of the Nursing Process, at least in theory, was widely accepted by both the education and management branches of nursing. One demonstration of this was the introduction of a new reporting system, which directed you towards considering patients' emotional, psychological and social state, as well as their physical condition. The forms for this replaced the old Kardex system, which certainly didn't provide this sort of direction and allowed for standard reporting one-liners like, 'Good day. Continued self-care', and 'Rather poorly. Pain relief given at 18.30.'

This new system wasn't especially welcomed. Some nurses thought that it would make them spend too much time writing – more bureaucracy! Others thought that it was trying to intellectualise the whole process of caring, which should actually be based on compassion and intuition rather than on clever words. These sentiments were strongly held. The result of this strong and widespread feeling was that two or three weeks after the introduction of the new system, if you'd looked at the nursing reports after a shift had gone home, you would have seen comments like, 'Good day. Continued self-care', and 'Rather poorly. Pain relief given at 18.30.' The few people who persisted in trying to write more were seen as 'essay writers' or 'airy fairy thinkers'. We had shifted back to report-writing that was mostly about physical aspects of patients' health and care.

Perhaps this example does no more than underline the notion of resistance to change in health care organisations (Stewart, 1989). But in fact this matches with the point I'm trying to make. If our profession has traditionally seen health in a certain sort of way, this will form part of our socialisation into professional values, reinforced by the 'hidden' curriculum; no matter how explicit 'formal' direction to think in other ways actually is, it will be very difficult to do so.

So despite the best efforts of policy makers and curriculum reformers, the 'hidden curriculum' continues to drive the formation of professional identities and professional values. And my argument is that within these are heavily embedded conceptions of the nature and value of health itself. This 'health' is more about disease absence than wider ideas of wellness. It is more about fixing 'broken machines' than understanding social contexts. It makes new or alternative perspectives on the idea of 'health' much harder to gather and sustain for the person struggling to study and understand the concept.

Turning Point?

A lot of my argument in this chapter has rested on the idea of professions powerfully instilling values. My claim has been that health care professions construct the identities of those seeking entry into them; and that part of this construction of identity involves assuming the values of the profession concerned. Moreover, as far as health

Turning Point? *continued*

studies goes, professions work with particular conceptions of health, generally revolving around the idea of health as 'disease absence'.

There is theoretical and empirical evidence for accepting both parts of this argument. With regard to the first – professions shaping identities-writers such as Merton *et al.* (1957) and Becker *et al.* (1977) present a picture of medical training in the USA, in which the profession strongly moulds the students trying to enter it. Nursing-related research, including that of Melia (1987) and Howkins and Ewens (1999) has also emphasised professions' power to determine the characters of their members and members-in-training.

But the difficulty with these kinds of accounts is the relative lack of power they allow to individual professionals and those learning to become professionals. It is as if these people are almost powerless to act in the face of the all-powerful determinism of the professional structure. There is no allowance for individual agency.

But this doesn't seem to correspond exactly with reality. While we need to acknowledge the power of professions and their capacity to mould professionals, it may be possible to make too much of these things. Individual professionals *do* challenge professional structures (Hart, 2004). This applies even to professionals in training, although perhaps the ways of doing so are subtle and covert. In a study of the professional socialisation of occupational therapy students, Clouder (2003) identified at least two ways in which the participants in her research established their own individual agency in the context of daunting professional structures. One was by 'learning to play the game'; that is to say, knowing what both the written and unwritten rules of the profession of occupational therapy were, of consciously 'putting up with things' or 'not rocking the boat' (Clouder, 2003: 217). Participants acted in these ways in order to progress through the system and although it could be argued that the balance of power remains very heavily with *structures*, to some extent at least these are being 'worked' by *individuals*. Arguably, progression through the system leads to a position where structural power can be more overtly challenged.

The other way Clouder identified students as establishing individual agency was through 'presentation of self' (Clouder, 2003: 218). This involved students making careful decisions about how they appeared and acted, and how they managed relationships with

Turning Point? *continued*

others. For example, it was thought to be wise not to 'clock watch', always to be willing to work just a little over the limit. Once more, while there is still considerable power being exercised by the structure, this is also a deliberate strategy on the part of individuals, giving a sense that they are not entirely helpless subjects determined by the professional system.

Perhaps reflection on our own professional lives and directions would lead us to the view that what is actually the case is that we 'take up a position somewhere between identification with an organisation and opposition to it' (Goffman, 1961: 280). We fall (or allow ourselves to fall) in between a point where our profession acts on us, and one where we act on our profession. But if that is the case, or if we allow more scope for individual agency than I did in my central argument, the questions at this particular Turning Point are, Do we use our individual capacity to help frame our understanding of the nature of the value of health? If we do, *how* do we use it? And *why* do we use it in that way?

What's gone on in this chapter?

I've described and discussed ways in which theorists have understood the nature of professions and of becoming a professional. The process of becoming a professional involves two things: learning what to do and how to do it; and learning what to believe and what to value. Professional values are intrinsic values. They are fundamental to professional identity. Our acquisiton of them emerges through a heady and difficult process of 'professional socialisation'. It's consequently very hard to resist, reject or challenge them. Beliefs about the nature of the value of health are central to the socialisation of health care professionals. We are encouraged to think of health in objectivist ways, revolving around the idea of it being 'absence of disease'. This makes it very hard to develop or critically appraise alternative conceptions of health, and so constitutes the second aspect of my argument for 'the difficulty of health studies'.

3 Disciplines, Diversity and Health Studies

What is this chapter going to do?

I move on in this chapter to the third aspect of my argument for 'the difficulty of health studies'. Academic disciplines claim to offer us new and important insights on 'health' and its nature. But there are problems with the application of disciplines to the study of health. Academic disciplines are not necessarily fixed, stable and indisputable bodies of knowledge. They contain ideologies, beliefs and values, and are highly vulnerable to pressures from the wider social world. Identifying these aspects of disciplines is hard. It is especially problematic if we are involved in the interdisciplinary study of health, and confront multiple values-based discourses.

Health and Academic Disciplines

So far in the development of my argument for 'the difficulty of health studies', I've made use of literature from a range of academic disciplines or sub-disciplines. These have included physiology, epidemiology, history, philosophy, sociology and education. This suggests that a variety of academic disciplines have an interest in the concept of health and practices associated with the concept. There should be little surprise in this idea. Health, as I've argued, is a fundamentally important human value. The interest and involvement of academic disciplines in making sense of health is natural, given their social role of promoting knowledge and understanding.

It also seems clear that the study of health can't be the preserve of just one academic discipline. Part of the account I've so far offered has built up a picture of 'health' that shifts according to individual perceptions, according to professional persona and values, and also according to social context. A single disciplinary perspective just wouldn't be able to capture and make sense of this complexity. Of course, particular perspectives have been (and continue to be) trumpeted over others. The project of 'medical imperialism' that I discussed earlier, for example, critiqued by David Armstrong and others involves the assertion that a set of academic disciplines (the physical sciences) can provide all the answers we need to the problems of illness and health. Academics from other disciplines, too, have tried to make claims for the special worth of their discipline's insights. For example, David Seedhouse writes in the preface to a collection of pieces analysing health reform policies in a number of different countries at the end of the twentieth century:

> Philosophical questions must be addressed if health reform is to be explored in any depth. (Seedhouse, 1995: ix)

Such attempts to vaunt on behalf of particular disciplines are understandable. Academics working in disciplines have been trained to engage in argument, and the most fundamental reason for arguing is that you believe in whatever position you are claiming (Bonnett, 2001). If you were a philosopher, say, it would seem strange if you didn't believe that the insights of philosophy were important for understanding the nature of health. But in another and quite fundamental way, attempts to assert particular disciplinary understandings appear wrong-headed, given what we know about health. It seems much more sensible to adopt the position described by Jennie Naidoo and Jane Wills:

> Health Studies. . . . draws on theoretical perspectives from a wide range of fields. . . . [We set out] to explore the diversity of those perspectives, illustrating the many ways in which health may be studied and how ideas from different disciplines contribute to our understanding of 'health'. (Naidoo and Wills, 2001: 1)

The term used by Naidoo and Wills for their exploration is 'interdisciplinary', to convey a sense of their moving between disciplines in order to bring those disciplines together and so develop stronger conceptions of health and the nature of health-related practices:

> The value of Health Studies is that, by drawing on many disciplines, it can provide a fuller account of health and begin to challenge existing boundaries of knowledge that lead to partial understandings of health. (Naidoo and Wills, 2001: 2)

Again, this position seems a sensible one. But while there are good reasons for taking an interdisciplinary approach to the study of health (this book is itself founded on a belief in the worth of such an approach), there is also a need to take a step back and consider whether it might also involve problems. There appears to be an assumption on the part of Naidoo and Wills, as well as others (e.g., Bunton and Macdonald, 2002) that an interdisciplinary approach is without difficulty. My argument now, though, is that interdisciplinary study can't be taken for granted as being uncomplicated. The idea of multiple academic disciplines contributing to the study of health is something that in itself needs to be considered, partly because within it might actually lie a further reason for 'the difficulty of health studies'.

What is a Discipline?

When we talk about 'disciplines', what do we mean? The Oxford Dictionary offers the following definitions:

> Training that produces obedience, self-control or a particular skill. . . . Controlled behaviour produced by such training. . . . A branch of instruction or learning. (Oxford University Press, 1983: 181)

These definitions are interesting and important because they start to extend our understanding of a discipline beyond it being simply 'a branch of instruction or learning'. Involvement in academic disciplines also entails:

Training and the development of particular skills. An academic – a philosopher, say – undergoes a long period of training, which is partly about developing understanding of the *content* of her discipline (the great philosophers, their theories and so on). But in order to develop that understanding, she also has to be trained to develop the skills required for her to produce her own insights (rigorous thinking, the capacity for sustained application to academic tasks, the ability to communicate in writing and otherwise, and so on). We might regard this as training in academic *processes.*

Controlled behaviour. Our philosopher can't develop her own insights unless she is able to exercise self-control to the extent that she can gather and examine arguments, synthesise and criticise them. She will get nowhere in the writing of her book on the philosophy of health, say, unless she has a well-honed self-control that moves her to her desk to write every morning rather than to the tennis court or the shops.

Obedience. This sounds rather severe, but again our philosopher won't make progress in her discipline unless she agrees to conform to certain rules. At a narrow level, in writing her insightful book she needs to obey the conventions of the discipline with regard to referencing and the presentation of arguments. At a broader level, she needs to conform to ways of relating her own arguments to those of others. This isn't to say that she is totally constrained – there has to be some creativity after all – but nor can she fly completely off the wall. If she didn't demonstrate at least some obedience to the conventions of her discipline, it's likely that the discipline itself would reject her insights.

So it doesn't seem too strong to talk about development in an academic discipline as 'training' and of this yielding certain sets of skills, along with the capacity for self-control in the application of these skills. As it happens, my own initial academic training was in the discipline of philosophy and my experience of this was as demanding as my slightly later experience of nursing (although in a very different kind of way). I wouldn't hesitate to call the experience of nursing I described in the previous chapter as *training*. Equally I wouldn't hesitate to talk of my time in a university philosophy department as training, too. If a discipline 'involves an ordered area or field of study' (Macdonald and Bunton, 2002: 17), then it seems sensible to imagine that we need to be inducted into particular ways of working so we can understand the nature of the order and our role in contributing to it.

Thinking Point

This characterisation of academic disciplines as areas of ordered study, requiring systematic training to understand and progress within them is commonly represented in some attitudes towards learning in higher education:

'Students' minds are empty containers waiting to be filled';
'Education is to sharpen that tool which is the mind'.

But this representation conflicts with another way of understanding the purpose of learning and education – one in which these things are seen as processes of growing and changing, rather than confining and defining (Marshall and Rowland, 1988: 16).

Thinking Point *continued*

How would you characterise your own experience of study in relation to health? Has it been a confining and defining experience, or a growing and changing one? What contributes to one or other of these kinds of experiences? If your experience has been both confining *and* changing (as it might well have been), how do you manage the conflict (or how can you manage it)?

The 'Health-Related Disciplines'

I've already suggested that a wide range of disciplines or sub-disciplines actually or potentially have an interest in the study of health. I've mentioned some that have played a part in my own arguments so far: physiology, epidemiology, history, philosophy, sociology and education. A quick survey of a few recent texts that one way or another address the area of health studies reveals a number of further disciplines or sub-disciplines that might contribute to understanding (Edmondson and Kelleher, 2000; Naidoo and Wills, 2001; Bunton and Macdonald, 2002.) These include psychology, social policy, economics, organisation and management, cultural studies and biomedicine.

It is certainly possible to engage in discussion about the contribution of these disciplines and sub-disciplines to understanding of the nature of health and health-related practices. We could, for example, consider whether they ought to be regarded as *primary* or *secondary* contributory disciplines. This is a distinction drawn by Bunton and Macdonald (2002), who argue that the development of theory and practice related to the *improvement* of health has depended on a number of 'primary feeder disciplines' (psychology, education, epidemiology and sociology). A number of 'secondary feeder disciplines' (including social policy, politics and ethics) have made important but lesser contributions (Bunton and Macdonald, 2002: 2).

In the same chapter, Bunton and Macdonald also refer to medical science as an 'underlying and pervasive influence' on health improvement-related thinking and practice (Bunton and Macdonald, 2002: 2). Interestingly, while they see it as having such influence, they decline to see it as a 'primary' (or even 'secondary') 'feeder discipline' for thought and practice on health improvement. But someone else might well take a different view. If they have a strong belief in the value

45

and efficacy of medicine, they will of course identify the physical sciences (including medical science) as fundamentally important in understanding and working for the improvement of health. So Jones (2000), for example, points to the 'medical model' as the impetus for certain sorts of health promotion-related theory and practice.

There is, then, a distinct possibility that what drives our choices about the disciplinary perspectives important to us in understanding 'health' is what we *already* know about the concept. Given this, there is also then the possibility that we go to a particular discipline whatever it is (philosophy, say), because it seems to have affinity with our own beliefs and values. These possibilities lead to two questions:

▸ Can we justify particular disciplinary focuses in our study of health over and above others? If so, how?
▸ To what extent do the disciplines contributing to health studies themselves hold particular beliefs and values?

I will consider the first of these questions in Chapter 4. At the moment, I want to concentrate on the second question.

Disciplines and Beliefs

Perhaps there is a tendency as we confront the might of the academic enterprise to be rather overawed by it. All this knowledge! What huge amounts of eminent understanding! The academic disciplines I've referred to and made use of so far (philosophy, sociology and so on) might take on the appearance of immutable canons.

Part of this possible sense of overawe in the presence of academic disciplines might emerge from the kinds of descriptions within the definition I started this discussion with. Such words as 'obedience. . . . self-control. . . . skill. . . . instruction. . . . learning' might well inspire concern. We may quite likely feel intimidated! The idea of academic disciplines as guardians of incontrovertible truth is also partly one put forward by academics themselves:

> It would be realistic to assume that the expression 'scientific research' would quickly bring the association 'incontrovertible fact' to the minds of members of a scientific community. (Giorgi, 1985: vii)

In talking of a 'scientific community', Giorgi means a community of those involved in the *physical* sciences. But as he goes on to suggest (although not necessarily to agree with), at least some in the *social* sciences actively seek the kind of association he speaks of, too. (And of course many of the disciplines that contribute to the study of 'health' are located in one or other of the physical or social sciences.) So the end product of our awed regard for academic disciplines, combined with the message they put out themselves, is very likely to lead us to believe that they contain solid bodies of knowledge, founded on stable ontology and epistemology.

I argue, though, that this view is mistaken. Far from solidity and stability, academic disciplines (even in the supposedly completely objective arena of the physical sciences) are subject to shifts in beliefs about what they can know and how they can know it. There are two reasons for making this claim:

▸ Simply because the *traits* of disciplines (self-control, obedience and so on) are so clear and apparently incontrovertible doesn't mean that the end *goal* of disciplinary study is equally clear;
▸ Academic disciplines, and academics, are part of the social world and as vulnerable to its pressures and changes as anyone or anything else.

I will explain each of these reasons a little more.

Academic Disciplines: Traits and Goals

The implications of the definitions and descriptions of academic disciplines discussed so far suggest that those involved move in a particular direction towards a fixed body of knowledge. But just because the *traits* of disciplines are so clear, we don't then have to believe that the *goals* of disciplinary study are equally clear. There is no necessary relationship of form between traits and goals here. Certainly it's possible – a requirement, in fact – for us to exercise the traits I've mentioned in our pursuit of knowledge, but this doesn't mean that we will meet (or will want to meet) an unchanging goal. In fact, the relationship between particular processes and particular goals isn't of this kind at all.

Let's take an example. Say I get it in my head that I want to become good at creative writing. I start going to evening classes on the subject. I get up early in the morning and stay up late to practice what I'm taught. I read the published work of notable creative writers. I begin to develop my own style. I start getting up even earlier and go to bed later still. I have done all this despite the fact I know that inherently I am a lazy person. I have developed and exercised (been encouraged to develop and exercise) the trait of self-discipline. I have practised obedience to the goal of better creative writing. But this still doesn't mean that the goal is *fixed*. I might be writing poetry or novels or TV plays. It doesn't even mean that I am writing according to a certain style. I could be writing experimentally, or I could be writing according to the principles of best-selling fiction. All that I've actually done is to learn to write better, to understand the process of writing more effectively. The goal of this process is unfixed, changing and flexible.

The same applies if I try and follow the path of self-control towards understanding a particular academic discipline. Certainly if I do so, I will begin, I hope, to understand the discipline better. But by itself, this *process* of self-understanding doesn't tell me anything about the actual *nature* of the discipline being studied itself, about the knowledge it contains or the truth of the claims it makes.

Academic Disciplines and the Wider Social World

There is sometimes a tendency to believe that academics are in some fashion removed from society; that they get on with their tasks of knowledge-making and understanding independently from the rest of us. They influence and shape *us*, but we don't (we can't) do the same to *them* (Chalmers, 1982).

But this simply doesn't make sense. However much they may like to believe otherwise, physiologists, epidemiologists, philosophers and sociologists all live in the real world. All academics do. They have to make money and spend money. They have to deal with other people. Many of them at one time or another have had to get up in the middle of the night to change babies' nappies! In other words, they live under the same political, economic, social and cultural influences as everybody else does. Bertrand Russell writes of philosophers (but I argue that his point applies to all academics):

> Philosophers are both effects and causes: effects of their social circumstances and of the politics and institutions of their time; causes (if they are fortunate) of beliefs which mould the politics and institutions of later ages. (Russell, 1979: 7)

This idea of the strong interrelationship between academics and wider society seems much more reasonable and acceptable than the notion that they are removed from everybody else. After all, if they are separated from the rest of society, what can they really tell us about our lives and ourselves? And why should we accept a remote but influencing source? If, though, we agree (as I argue that we have to) with the idea of the profound interrelationship between academics and society, we can't at the same time believe that academic disciplines remain unchanged and unchanging, not subject to wider social beliefs about their spheres of knowledge. They must be both influencing and influenced.

Ethics provides us with an example of disciplinary change as a result of broader social and political influence. The late eighteenth century, as I've already discussed, was the period of The Enlightenment, a time of relatively rapid scientific advancement in which many discoveries were made about the nature of man and the physical world. A general belief emerged that it was possible to continue making these discoveries almost without limit through the application of scientific, rational thought. The German philosopher Immanuel Kant (1724–1804), for example, tried to apply principles of rationality to the development of rules about how we should behave – rules of ethics.

His proposal (Paton, 1948) was that while we live in a world subject to the natural laws of causation, we still retain freedom of will and have the capacity because of this to act morally, or otherwise. So our ethical choices must be framed within an independent reality. Reason exists within this independent reality and the right use of reason is directed towards ethical ends. Reason demands that we act out of duty for its own sake. Thus ethical actions are those which obey universally held principles of duty – or which as rational beings we can will to become universal principles. In other words, as a rational being with obligations to other rational beings, there *just are* some ethical rules I must follow. This kind of duty-based theory is often referred to as one of deontology.

Kant's deontological theory was founded on the belief that rationality (the cornerstone of the Enlightenment) provided the key to understanding and explaining the nature of ethical action. It can clearly be seen as a product of its social times. Equally, it is possible to see what many regard as an opposing ethical theory – Utilitarianism – as rooted in *its* own times. Utilitarianism's most famous advocate was John Stuart Mill (1806–1873). The theory of Utilitarianism proposes that in considering the ethical worth of a particular action, what should motivate us is not certain irrevocable duties. Rather, we should be guided by a concern for the *consequences* of our actions – especially the degree to which happiness will accrue as a result of performing the action (Mill, 1962).

Mill developed his ethics of consequences in the mid-nineteenth century, a time when trade and commerce were key and when populations (at least in Britain and parts of Europe) were becoming urbanised. People became dependent, as never before, on others who might actually be physically far removed from them. For example, a town-dweller's well-being would depend substantially on distant companies who supplied their everyday need for water and for sewage disposal. So the development of ethical theory based on thought about the impact and consequences of action, in as wide a sphere as possible becomes understandable. Once again, theory development and social context connect to each other.

It can therefore be argued that two quite different theories of ethics sprang up from different social, political and economic times. My claim is not that the purpose of ethics, in the broadest sense, changed between the emergence of deontology and the rise of consequentialist theory such as utilitarianism. Its concern with examining the worth or value of conduct stayed constant, and in fact endures into our own times (Duncan, 2001). However, the discipline (or sub-discipline, as ethics is one of three main branches of philosophy) has changed. It has changed because new theory has developed as a result of altering social times. Emerging theory has to take account of existing theory. Modification, amendment or possibly rejection takes place. The sub-discipline is no longer the same.

Thinking Point

Chapter 8 will discuss in more detail the impact of disciplinary change on the critical perspectives on health offered by ethics. For now, though, consider the two ethical theories briefly outlined above – one deontological and the other consequentialist. How might your own perspective on the nature of health and the purpose of health care shift as a result of considering one theory, and then the other?

What I've just focused on is the idea that academic disciplines are not neutral and immovable bodies of knowledge but in fact are, to a large extent, products of their social times. The theories and practices they contain change and develop. This idea of disciplinary change has itself been theorised by a number of important thinkers, in particular the philosopher of science Thomas Kuhn. While Kuhn's theory was originally developed to explain progress in the physical sciences, it has also been influential in shaping thinking (as well as provoking argument) across a wider field, including the social sciences (Macdonald and Bunton, 2002). Kühn proposes (1962, 1970) that there are three basic stages in scientific development:

- First a *pre-paradigm* stage, in which a number of theories compete for supremacy ('paradigm' can be understood as a way of seeing and interpreting the world, or an aspect of the world);
- Second, a period of what he calls *normal science*, during which the dominant theory is widely accepted and worked with;
- Third a *crisis* stage, in which the dominant theory is challenged and replaced by another.

Of course, not everyone engaged in academic work and discovery is actively involved in trying to shift and change the paradigms according to which disciplines operate. Most people (as in lots of other areas of life) are quite happy to rub along and work according to the dominant paradigm (Magee, 1975). But the point is that paradigms do compete and shift. The nature of academic disciplines does change. The idea of disciplines as stable, unaltering bodies of knowledge with which I began this section doesn't, on reflection, seem quite so realistic. If this alternative account that I've developed is accepted, then it seems reasonable to reach the conclusion that disciplinary shift and alterations entail changing beliefs and values. Ontology and epistemology can be challenged. The orthodoxy can be embraced or rejected.

Academic Disciplines: The Challenge for Health Studies

It's important to be clear about the shifting and altering nature of academic disciplines, because it poses a particular problem for the study of health. As I've already said, some writers seem to believe that the study of health through particular academic disciplines, or in an interdisciplinary way, is relatively unproblematic. Interdisciplinarity, in fact, is often seen as a positive benefit. Edmondson and Kelleher, for example, talk of using an interdisciplinary approach to explore 'sources of creative tension' (Edmondson and Kelleher, 2000: 4) between disciplines. But there are also difficulties with the study of health through the lens of a particular discipline or disciplines, and unless we understand what these are, there seems little possibility of generating, let alone using, any 'creative tension'. I argue that academic disciplines pose a challenge for the study of health in three ways:

▸ There is in the first place the problem of making sense of any given discipline that might contribute to health studies;
▸ There is second the difficulty of trying to engage in *interdisciplinary* study of health.
▸ Finally, there is the problem of the shifting context in which disciplinary or interdisciplinary study takes place.

I will examine each of these difficulties in turn.

Health Studies – Making Sense of Disciplines

I've suggested that academic disciplines form ordered areas of study; they develop the capacity and skills that enable someone to acquire knowledge and understanding related to a given area. But the area itself is subject to shifts in beliefs about what can be known and how such knowledge can be gained, as well as to how knowledge should be used. This creates a complex picture of the nature of a discipline. The complexity shows itself in a number of ways.

First, there may be competing ideologies about the purpose of the discipline. For example, if we think of the discipline of education, what is the purpose of understanding more about education? Is it so that we become better able to train or mould according to some kind of economic specification demanded by society? Or is it so that we become better at helping people to develop their own self-awareness and capacity, regardless of any economic requirement on the part of society (Peters, 1973)? These two different views of the purpose in developing educational understanding will yield two quite separate academic projects.

Second, those involved in academic disciplines engage in a number of different kinds of discourse to promote their understanding of the discipline's purpose. (From Marshall and Rowland, 1998: 32, I understand 'discourse' to mean the language, vocabulary and methods used by an academic discipline to develop and present its arguments.) They may engage in the construction of *normative* or *analytical* theory or argumentation. They may also use argument based on *empirical evidence*.

Thinking Point

▶ *Normative* theory and argumentation attempts to argue or theorise on the basis of prescribed norms or standards that have already been assumed (Lacey, 1976). For example, I might construct an argument for viewing 'health' as a good, in which certain norms have already been assumed, such as 'one ought to be healthy'.

▶ *Analytic* theory and argumentation tries to explain how and why something is the way it is (Bonnett, 2001). So I might construct an argument for 'health' being seen as a good by examining the component parts of the idea of 'health' (physical functioning enabling participation in social life, and so on).

▶ An argument based on *empirical evidence* employs data collected through observation in some way of actual phenomena or events in the real world (say, through interviews or questionnaires). So in my argument for health as a good, I might use empirical data to support a particular understanding of the nature of 'health' – that it is, for example, the 'absence of disease' (Tones and Green, 2004). In this way, I could assert (because disease absence is generally considered to be a good thing) that 'health' is therefore a good.

Of course, it is possible to combine normative and analytical theory and argumentation, and argumentation using empirical evidence. Consider my brief discussion above on the purposes of developing understanding about the nature of education. What might be the form of a normative, an analytical and an empirically-based argument in favour of *health education*, founded on one or other (or both) conceptions of the purpose of education?

The aim of this 'Thinking Point' is to encourage you to recognise that disciplinary argument is likely to be complex and multilayered. It involves different kinds of theorising and argumentation, all overlain by separate senses of the discipline's purpose. The challenge posed by an academic discipline to those studying health is to make sense of this complexity for the benefit of their own particular health-related focus. Moreover, those involved in health studies frequently don't have the benefit of training ('disciplining') in the area concerned. Academic disciplines and their discourses become understandable, at least in part, through such training. How can the health studies student make sense of it all?

Making Sense of the Interdisciplinary Study of Health

But the difficulty doesn't end there. I've argued that a broad range of academic disciplines has an interest in health as well as potentially contributing to our understanding of the concept. How do we get to grips with them all? More specifically, we need to be aware of, understand and interpret the competing ideologies of the separate disciplines. (This is as well as the requirement for understanding ideological competition *within* disciplines, which I have just discussed.)

The problem of interdisciplinary study is compounded by the fact that different disciplines hold not only separate ideological but also separate *conceptual* understanding. This emerges, of course, from their different ontological and epistemological beliefs and positions. But these differences are made confusing by the fact that quite often in disciplines connected to the study of health, separate conceptual understandings are masked by use of the *same language* to express what are actually *different concepts* (Creme and Lea, 1997). An example from the disciplines of philosophy and sociology will help to illustrate this.

Philosophy, and more particularly its branch of ethics, understands 'ethics' itself as enquiry into the nature of 'the good' and 'the right' (Lacey, 1976). As such, it is a *normative* project – ethicists are at least in part trying to justify their own understanding of what is good or worthwhile, an understanding they have already assumed; or they are attempting to critique another kind of (assumed) understanding. So for philosophers, 'ethics' centrally involves evaluative judgement and justification. But for sociology, standard use of the term 'ethics' does not entail evaluation or appraisal at all, except perhaps in an extremely wide and rather vague way. Most frequently for the sociologist, 'ethics' involves *description* of a particular ethical position adopted by certain individuals or groups. The sociologist describes ethical issues and the relationship between those issues and her or his conception of human society. He or she may even suggest that there is a need in a general sense for social understanding of the nature and purpose of ethics to change (Williams, 2003: 199–204). But this largely *descriptive* conception of 'ethics' is not the same as that of the philosopher who advocates and defends particular *normative* positions. This will give rise to very different kinds of discourses. The philosopher developing a discourse on, say, the ethics of health care would be trying to defend (or critique) particular ethical stances that it was assumed, say, would lead to better or worse health. The sociologist's discourse, on the other hand, would simply be trying to describe those stances and how and why they had emerged in the society concerned. (Although as I'll discuss in Chapter 9, this doesn't mean to say that this discourse is without underpinning – but perhaps not explicit – ideologies and values.)

Of course I'm not suggesting that one approach is less important than the other – the discourse of the philosopher and the sociologist can both be very helpful in developing our understanding of the nature of health. But there are two things that this example points up:

▸ If we are studying health in an interdisciplinary way, we need to be aware that *separate disciplines may be using the same words in quite different ways and for different purposes.*
▸ Second, it's possible that by virtue of our own disciplinary background or preferences *we may assume that others possess the same understanding as we do – and this may not be the case at all.*

There is, though, a further difficulty emerging from the interdisciplinary study of health. As I've already suggested, disciplines use a range of discourses to develop the understanding they offer and to promote their lines of argumentation. It's also reasonable to suggest that different disciplines have preferences with regard to the kind of discourse in which they engage, because there is a belief it advances disciplinary purpose. This certainly seems to be so with regard to the disciplines potentially contributing to an understanding of health. The physical sciences, such as physiology, frequently base their argumentation on empirical evidence (Cedar with Hubbard, 2001). This is also true to some extent with certain disciplines of the social sciences, such as psychology (Giorgi, 1985). These preferences, as I've already discussed, may have very little to do with searches for 'the truth' and much more to do with such things as pragmatic tactical alignment with powerful domains like medicine. In contrast with disciplines that seem to have a preference for empiricism, philosophy and its sub-discipline of ethics, for example, rely almost exclusively on normative or analytic argumentation (Duncan, 2001).

If we are likely to encounter this range of discourses in our interdisciplinary study of health, we need to recognise their separate purposes, their strengths and limitations, as well as their relationship to the purpose and nature of the discipline concerned (Powell, 1999). But we also need to be wary of interdisciplinary study leading to a confounding and potentially misleading fusion of discourses. We need to recognise the risk of certain kinds of discourse, with a particular purpose, turning into different kinds of discourse with another sort of purpose, all under the enthusiastically (and maybe uncritically)-held banner of 'interdisciplinary studies'. A result of this may be the development of *hidden discourses* potentially leading in turn to *confused conceptual understanding*. An example will help to illustrate what I mean.

One of the central ways in which psychology has been applied to health studies is to establish how and why people change their health behaviour – especially 'lifestyle' behaviour such as smoking, eating and drinking alcohol. Part of the task of health psychology is to examine health beliefs and thus offer predictors to how and why people will behave, given certain sets of circumstances and factors (Ogden, 2001). Over the latter half of the twentieth century and into the twenty-first, much attention has been given to the development of predictive models of health behaviour (see, e.g., Prochaska and DiClemente 1982, Becker, 1984; Tones and Green, 2004). A lot of this work has been based on empirical studies; attempts to establish what people believe about their health, and their reasons for engaging in particular health-related behaviours. To this extent, psychology's discourse on health beliefs and models of health behaviour can be seen as empirically based and analytic. (It is analytic because it uses the empirical evidence in part to explain how and why people engage in the health behaviours that they do.)

So far, all this seems justifiable. Frequently, though, something strange happens within this kind of health behaviour-related discourse. Take the Health Action Model (HAM), originally devised by Tones (1979, 1981). In a retrospective 'review' of his model (Tones and Green, 2004), Keith Tones and Jackie Green identify its sources – the range of health behaviour models and associated empirical work that preceded his own model. The key addition in his own model is a system that emphasises the importance of enabling factors, which together make up a 'supportive environment that makes "the healthy choice the easy choice" ' (Tones and Green, 2004: 79). Once more, up to this point we can probably see their argument as justifiable in the context of the empirical and analytic discourses they have represented. But now consider what comes next:

> An alternative way of expressing the importance of these enabling factors is to assert that *health promotion is charged with removing those psychological, behavioural and environmental barriers that militate against people making healthy choices*. (Tones and Green, 2004: 79–80, my italics)

Tones and Green for some reason have now converted an *empirical-analytic* argument into a *normative* one. They are arguing not only that this is how and why people change behaviour; but also that behaviour change towards 'health' is something that ought to be encouraged, and that the relevant authorities ought to take their responsibilities seriously in this regard.

My concern here isn't to question the *content* of Tones' and Green's argument. I'm not interested at the moment in seeking to agree or disagree with the stance that they are taking (the requirement for supportive environments and public agencies to enable behaviour change). I will consider more closely how this sort of position can be justified in Chapter 8. For the moment, I want simply to draw attention to the *process* in which they've engaged-their move from empirical-analytic argumentation to normative argumentation. (Argument intended to advance a position that is based on already assumed norms; in this case the idea that health and behaviour changes for health are good things.) There are two problems with this process:

▸ The writers haven't made clear what they are doing;
▸ The basis for their move is inadequate because no part of their previous argument has been concerned with justifying the normative assumptions they've now made explicit.

We need to try and understand what's gone on, and why.
There are, I think, good reasons for Tones and Green making the assumptions that they do. However, reasons for the assumptions need to be made more explicit if we are to avoid the feeling that something rather subversive is going on in this chapter. As they say (Tones and Green, 2004: 78), part of the purpose in constructing the HAM towards the end of the 1970s was to provide a theoretical basis to support what was then the emerging occupation of health promotion. Theory, as we've discussed, is frequently closely connected with ideology. Theory development is often undertaken to justify and promote a particular

ideological position, especially if it relates to purposes of policy or practice. So we could suggest that Tones was theorising health action in order to promote the ideology of health promotion, which in turn would assist the development of the occupation.

But realising this emphasises the fundamental difficulties that the possibility of 'hidden' discourses, represented by this example, pose for the interdisciplinary study of health:

▸ Because study is interdisciplinary, we will be encountering a range of discourses. Not necessarily grounded in one particular discipline, it may be hard for us to detect when moves from one kind of discourse to another have taken place and whether those moves are justifiable.

▸ Some, even many, 'health' academics and theorists are actively involved in interdisciplinary work and so move, perhaps unconsciously, between discourses. There is not necessarily an intention to 'hide' styles of argumentation, but it may be hard for us to keep up with the moves they make *just because* they are interdisciplinary.

▸ Because the study of health is often focused towards practical ends (becoming more skilled at improving health, or in understanding health care practices, say), there is every likelihood that the theory emerging through the discourses that we try and understand will be underpinned by a fair amount of ideology. So if the discourses are 'hidden', in some way, while there isn't necessarily any intention to deceive, it might actually look that way to us!

Thinking Point

I've identified two ways in which the interdisciplinary study of health might cause difficulties: the use of the same language by separate disciplines to express what are actually different concepts; and the application of 'hidden' discourses as we move back and forth between disciplines, potentially leading to confused conceptual understanding.

I've given examples related to both of these difficulties. From your experience and study of health, can you think of further examples? Can you think of other kinds of difficulties related to interdisciplinary study? (You might want to delve further back in your experience to consider this second question if, for example, you've engaged in previous interdisciplinary study – media studies, say, or studies of a particular society and culture such as American or European Studies.

The Shifting Context of Health-Related Disciplinary and Interdisciplinary Study

One of my central claims in this chapter has been that academics and academic disciplines are not in some mysterious way disconnected from society. In fact academic disciplines and society are fundamentally interrelated, with disciplinary development both shaping and shaped by the society in which the disciplines exist. From discussion in earlier chapters, a sense should also be developing that the broader context of health and health care is shifting and changing in important ways, too; for example, through the development of challenging, non-objectivist accounts of health, and 'new' methodologies for researching health. Nor are shifts in the context of health and health care confined to theory. Despite the resistance to change in practice that I discussed in Chapter 2, there is no doubt that new ways of thinking about what professionals need to do and how they need to do it are highly influential (Barr, 2002).

Shifts in health care practice encouraged or required by policy have revolved around the need to move from seeing clients and patients of health care professionals as simply *passive recipients* of care to much more *active consumers* (Department of Health, 1997, 2000). Some academic commentators on this process have theorised these trends in the context of so-called late modernity, an era in which *reflexiveness* is all-important. They have argued that the capacity of increasingly skilled and clever laypeople to use and manipulate systems has led to the layperson becoming not just a 'health consumer' but in fact a *quasi-producer* of health (Giddens, 1990; Williams, 2003).

All this raises essential issues for academic disciplines. On some accounts, the relationship between health care professional and client has changed beyond recognition. Professionals have moved (have had to move) towards seeing *people* rather than problems; people whose health is as much determined by their social context and environment as it is by their own personal actions. This move has been predicated, as I've already argued, by broader and more flexible notions of what we understand by 'health' in the first place (Cribb and Duncan, 2002). This then is the issue for those considering academic disciplines and the social context of health and health care:

▸ If the idea of the fundamental interrelationship between academic disciplines and wider social context is accepted, and if the social context of health care has changed profoundly as I've suggested, then surely academic disciplines with an interest in health and health care will have had to change, too?

I want to argue that this is true in at least some respects and as such creates further difficulty for those engaged in the study of health. In the first place, it's possible to note shifts in disciplines (or at least shifts in the centre of gravity of disciplines) as they attempt to take account and respond to the needs of the changing social context. If we look to psychology, for example, it's possible to detect the emergence of ways of thinking that attempt to marry the classic interests of psychology as a discipline (individual identity, behaviour and cognition) with the broader interests demanded by changes in the health and health care context. So the area of sociopsychology has emerged, relating these classic interests to such things as the place of society, institutions and organisations in shaping individual and community psychology (Tudor, 1996). Again, philosophy and more especially ethics has responded to the demands of the context through the emergence of bioethics, with its particular focus on the moral basis of health care and the ethical justification of health-related actions (Beauchamp and Childress, 1994). Among further examples, it's possible to point to the increased interest of sociology in not only explaining the social nature of health and sickness, and individuals' responses to these things; but also critiquing health and health care-related institutions and practices, often quite radically (Bunton, Nettleton and Burrows, 1995.)

I argue that to a great extent all of these shifts in academic disciplinary perspective and concern have taken place as a result of our unsettled and rapidly altering social times. Above them all, it could be said, but actually permeating the disciplines themselves, are overarching, changed and changing theoretical perspectives such as individualisation (Bourdieu, 1986), the risk society (Beck, 1992), consumerism (Gabe and Calnan, 2000) and postmodernism (Foucault, 1973). These are what Ball refers to as 'grand narratives' (Ball, 2003: 13).

There is, of course, the question of the nature of the relationship between shifting disciplines and changing society. Which is changing which? In a sense, if we accept the fundamental interconnection between the two, this question is of much less importance for the health studies student than the more practical one: *what does it all mean for me?*

I argue that the response to this question is twofold:

▸ First, if we accept this kind of analysis of shifting context and changing disciplines, there is a need for the health studies student to try and understand the theoretical and disciplinary shifts that are taking place. This is not necessarily an easy thing to do, given my previous arguments related to understanding disciplinary complexity and engaging in interdisciplinary study;

▸ Second, though, while this task of understanding might be difficult, it could well be very helpful to the health studies student in the long run. If changing academic disciplines represent changing society, and if changing perspectives on health is part of this mix, then studying the impact of disciplines on society (and *vice versa*) could be very helpful to us in understanding the nature of health itself.

Health Warning: The Need to Pause!

This warning is serious! If we are to make progress in dealing with the difficulty of health studies, now is the time to pause and take stock before deciding how to move on. The pause certainly isn't a defeat. After all, I hope that by now you have a clear idea of the nature of the difficulty in studying health. And understanding this difficulty is the first and most crucial step in deciding how to deal with it.

My account of 'the difficulty of health studies' in these beginning chapters has involved the following:

▸ Both objectivist and interpretivist accounts of health cause problems for the health studies student. The objectivist account ('health as the absence of disease', say) just doesn't seem to say enough about a complex concept. Interpretivist accounts (for example, health as 'the foundations for achievement') perplex us because in order to have very much meaning, they need to have limits imposed on them. But what are those limits?

▸ The common sense middle position ('health is disease absence but it might well be more than this, too') is problematic, particularly for health care professionals. This is because of the ways in which the ideologies, beliefs and values inculcated within them through their professional training and background move professionals towards particular ways of understanding the nature of the value of health.

▸ The academic disciplines that supposedly offer us illumination of the problems associated with understanding health and health care are themselves filled with ideologies, beliefs and values.

Approaching these (often without the benefit of a lengthy formal training in the discipline concerned) poses difficulties for the student of health, who may well be attempting to grapple with multiple disciplinary perspectives.

In sum, 'the difficulty of health studies' is substantial. But it is not insurmountable. With the understanding of the nature of the problem that I hope we've gathered so far, I want now to move to considering how to deal with it. I want to start building, if you like, an agenda for tackling the difficulty of studying health.

Turning Point?

I have talked in this chapter of the distinctive nature of academic disciplines, of the need for what I've sometimes called 'training' to understand their purposes and discourses and of the consequent problem of studying health in an interdisciplinary way. It is certainly very important to make these points because they present very real problems for the study of health. In this Turning Point, however, I want briefly to discuss a way of generally thinking about health studies that might move us towards ways of understanding and working which help cross disciplinary divides.

In an earlier 'Thinking Point', I mentioned areas of interdisciplinary study that you might have been engaged in before coming to the study of health – Media Studies, for example, or European Studies. The trend towards gathering a number of academic disciplines together and applying them to examination of a particular area has been an important one in higher education in recent times. So too has been the idea of taking a particular discipline or sub-discipline (for example, ethics) and 'applying' it in a range of other disciplinary contexts (Illingworth, 2004). Among the reasons for this latter trend is recognition of the need, given that undergraduate level education is now a pre-requisite for entry into the professions, for all educated at degree level to hold certain kinds of competencies. Can you think of other possible reasons for the emergence of 'applied' disciplinary thinking?

In general, it might be possible to construct an argument for divisions between academic disciplines becoming less in recent years, although I would continue to argue as I have done for the difficulty of interdisciplinary study in the context of health. However, these

Turning Point? *continued*

trends and developments might provide us with a 'way into' working across disciplinary divides.

Creme and Lea (1997: 27), arguing from the viewpoint that academic disciplinary divisions are now much less clear than they have been, assert that in approaching the task of academic learning (and particularly writing), much depends on particular orientations of courses and degree programmes. The way students are required to study and write depends on these orientations. There may in fact be several different orientations within a single degree programme:

> For example, you may find yourself studying issues concerning the environment from a geographical, social, cultural or biological perspective, depending upon the particular course or unit you are taking. (Creme and Lea, 1997: 27–28)

This leads them to the idea of *fields of study*. Rather than concentrating on one discipline, with its particular discourses and conventions, students should be prepared to think of using different disciplines that together contribute to the particular field of study – in our case, health. Doing this requires thinking (and writing) in different ways, according to the separate disciplines contributing to the field of study. So in studying health, we might be called on to analyse quantitative epidemiological data. We might be asked to comment on the validity of the methodology employed in a particular psychological study. Again, a lecturer might ask you to offer a reflective piece on a 'critical incident' you've been exposed to in your professional lives, in which you analyse what happened, why it happened and how it might have been different.

We might well be prepared to accept the idea of health as a *field of study*. There seem to be good reasons to do so, given what we now know about the nature of health and what we need to take into account to move towards understanding it more critically and deeply. If this is the case, there seem to be two major requirements being made of us:

› The need *to be prepared* to think in a range of different ways;
› The need to be *able to respond* to the requirement to think in a range of ways (e.g., through assignments and assessments).

Turning Point? *continued*

In turn, I want to pose two questions:

▸ Do you agree that we should be seeking to regard 'health' as a field of study? If so, why? If not, why not?

▸ If we do accept the idea of 'health' as a field of study, and so the need to prepare ourselves for a range of different ways of thinking and to be able to respond to these, how might we go about equipping ourselves for these demands?

It would be helpful to think about these questions before moving onto the next chapter.

What's gone on in this chapter?

I have reviewed and discussed the nature of academic disciplines, particularly focusing on the idea that they are stores of ideologies, beliefs and values. As students of health, there is a need to recognise this, but doing so may be difficult because we don't necessarily have extensive training in the discipline whose particular insights we feel might be useful to us. The nature of health also means that we are likely to have to engage in examination of a number of disciplines, each with their particular ways of engaging in discourse. Understanding 'multiple discourses' (the requirement of interdisciplinary study) is likely to be especially problematic. Finally, I discussed the impact of the shifting context of health on academic disciplines concerned with understanding the concept – and the requirement of health studies students to try and understand the effect of one on the other.

4 Developing an Agenda for Studying Health

What is this chapter going to do?

I've now established the three components of 'the difficulty of health studies': competing ontological and epistemological disputes; professional ideologies, beliefs and values feeding these; and academic disciplinary diversity making it hard to get to grips with discourses on health. This chapter sets out an agenda for tackling these components, and thus the overall difficulty. I argue that we need to engage in processes of both critical *analysis* and critical *reflection* in order to address the difficulty. We need to be analytic because many of the arguments we encounter are ostensibly presented as rational and analytic themselves. We need to be reflective because underlying so much of the field of health studies are beliefs and values – including our own – which can only be properly understood through examination extending beyond simply the rational. My agenda proposes using critical analysis and critical reflection to examine the use and worth of a small number of disciplinary discourses related to the concept of health and the practice of health care.

Where to Begin? Dangling Threads, Faucets and Philosophers!

A major concern in trying to tackle the difficulty of studying health is quite simply the one of knowing where to begin. Reviewing my arguments for the nature of the difficulty, it's possible to identify a whole raft of issues and questions, some relatively small-scale and others seemingly fundamental. How do we start to get to grips with them? How do we pick up all these dangling threads?

Thinking Point

Skim-read through the first three chapters again, trying to pick out what seem the key issues and questions raised in relation to 'the difficulty of health studies'. List these key issues and questions, keeping them to one side as you read this chapter. When you've finished reading the chapter, look at your own list and consider whether the issues and questions that you raised yourself are matched by my interpretation. If there is a gap between your own list and my interpretation, it might be worth asking yourself why this is so.

My intention now is to try and develop a kind of agenda for the rest of the book that will try and tie up at least some of these threads. My plan is briefly to return to what I think are the central problems that have been raised for the study of health so far and then to set out my ideas on how it might be possible to tackle the problems. I will finish the chapter by mapping out the shape of the rest of the book. I will also discuss a particular question about its direction that may be troubling you at this point. This is the place of biomedicine in my direction and argument.

One thing I want to make clear is that this chapter, and the rest of the book, *don't* provide definitive and clear-cut answers to all the problems that have emerged. Quite possibly the book won't provide straightforward answers to even just some of these problems. What I want to do is to try and encourage, and to suggest ways of developing, *clearer thinking* (and so, hopefully, *better understanding*) in relation to the highly elusive concept of health.

I'm not at all certain that definitive answers to the problems raised actually exist. There have certainly been many assertions by academics (and others) that they've come up with 'the answers' to health studies-related problems. Look again, for example at Chapter 1 and the clarity with which JG Scadding (1988) concludes his argument for viewing health as 'the absence of disease'. But the appearance of counter-argument and the persistence of debate make it reasonable to think the original 'answers' aren't quite as complete as they might first have appeared.

The American philosopher Elmer Sprague (1978) describes an occasion when he had a leaky faucet (tap) in his apartment in Brooklyn.

He apparently called a plumber who came and mended it and told him it was possible the problem would recur. The philosopher wasn't to worry though, the plumber said, because Sprague could easily fix the problem himself. There was no need to call him again – he would show Sprague how to do it himself. When the plumber had shown the philosopher what to do, he turned and said with a tone of mild warning in his voice, 'But don't fix it too good.'

Sprague was writing in a preface to his book on metaphysics, a book dealing with what we might consider the 'big' philosophical questions, such as the nature of time and space and the existence of God. His intention was to let his readers know that these kinds of 'big' problems shouldn't be 'fixed too good' either, partly because they weren't amenable to such fixing and partly because if somebody tried, they'd be bound to get the fixing wrong. With this story of plumbers and philosophers in mind, I want to say that I can't (and I won't try to) fix the difficulty of health studies 'too good'. But I hope that the exploration and discussion this agenda-setting chapter is going to plot will be good enough to enable clearer thinking and better understanding.

Return to the Central Problems: Content and Process

Sorting through the threads that the first three chapters have left dangling, there is a need to identify again the three central 'difficulties of health studies' from which it seems that many of the others stem. It's also important to recognise once more that each of these difficulties is very closely connected to the others. My argument now is that, in broad terms, each of these difficulties has a *content* aspect to it; and each a *process* aspect.

Thinking Point

When I talk of a difficulty having a *process* aspect to it, I mean that part of the problem relates to what we need to do, actions or operations we need to undertake, in order to understand the difficulty more fully and be better able to deal with it.

In talking of a difficulty having a *content* aspect, I mean that there is something *in the nature of the problem itself* that makes it demanding of our time and attention.

An example might help to support this distinction between content and process. I have deliberately chosen a 'non-health' example for the time being so that the actual process/ content distinction is as clear as possible. The game of chess presents an overall difficulty to the person learning to play it. This is the difficulty of how to win your games! Within this difficulty is a *process* aspect and a *content* one. The process aspect is developing the knowledge and understanding that will enable you to move your pieces in the appropriate way before you actually sit down to a game (e.g., knowing that pawns can move two squares to begin with and only one thereafter, bishops move diagonally and so on). The content aspect is making these moves in ways that will enable you to win in a particular game, against a certain opponent who is skilled and making moves and counter-moves as clever as your own.

Of course in this example and many others, while the distinction between process and content aspects of a difficulty can be made clear, there is a heavy degree of connection between the two – a reliance of one on the other. Presumably, someone wouldn't even contemplate tackling the *process* aspect of the difficulty unless they were serious about engaging with the *content* aspect and ultimately tackling the overall difficulty of winning games – because this is at least partly why you learn to play chess! Content aspects of difficulties feed process ones – it is hard to learn to play chess skilfully and to the level that you can win games because the overall 'problem' (winning) is so hard (assuming your opponent is as skilful as or even more skilled than you).

Try and think now of an example from your own personal life or professional practice of a difficulty that involves both process and content aspects. Try and think as clearly as possible about what the process difficulty actually is and what is the content difficulty. How does one connect to the other?

Although the study of health is much, much messier than chess (I would argue), I believe that in a similar way process and content aspects of 'the difficulty of health studies' are profoundly connected. We need to understand both aspects of each of the component difficulties of health studies that I've so far identified in order to understand properly the nature of the overall difficulty – and so be able to deal with it. Here again is each of the component difficulties identified in the first three chapters:

Competing ontological and epistemological accounts of 'health'. What is the nature of health? Given this nature, what are we able to know about it? How can we know it? How do we decide between the accounts on offer?

The impact of professional beliefs and values on our conceptions of health. Our thoughts about the nature of health are heavily influenced by the beliefs and value that our professional training and education inculcate within us. This is one important reason why a seemingly sensible 'middle position' on the nature of health (absence of disease, but also allowing a degree of interpretation beyond this) might be hard to adopt.

Attempting to understand academic disciplinary discourses related to health. The difficulty here is not only trying to understand the discourse of a particular discipline but also (given what we've already discovered about the problematic nature of the concept of health) trying to operate in an interdisciplinary way. It seems right to think that we need multiple critical perspectives if we are going to move towards reasoned and proper understanding of the concept. But given the nature of academic disciplines, and given the 'shifting context' in which both academics and those interested in their ideas work, achieving understanding through disciplinary and interdisciplinary examination could well prove difficult.

I want now to develop a slightly more detailed account of the process and content aspects within each of these component difficulties of the overall 'difficulty of health studies'.

The Difficulty of Competing Ontological and Epistemological Accounts of Health: Content and Process

It seems relatively clear to *identify* the content aspect of this difficulty, although *dealing* with it appears much less certain. We know that there are certain ontological arguments for the nature of health and that they can broadly be classified as objectivist ('health' as some kind of objective, discoverable reality); and interpretivist (what we mean by 'health' depends on individual interpretation and understanding of particular context). These separate ontological positions lead in turn to distinct epistemological ones. Broadly, the objectivist believes that we can investigate 'health' within the positivist paradigm and in applying quantitative methodologies we will make perfectly adequate discoveries. The interpretivist, on the other hand, argues that investigation needs to employ qualitative methodologies, attempting to elicit individual understanding (although as I discussed in Chapter 1, limits might be set on that understanding).

The *content* challenge within all this is to recognise and analyse these separate positions. From this analysis, it should be possible to justify (or refute) a particular position. Perhaps it might even be possible to reconcile them. The *process* challenge is to try and work out what is going on beneath the surface, so to speak, in relation to each of the positions. In particular, there is a need to recognise that positions have been assumed at least in part because of underlying ideologies. We need not only to recognise but also to chart and understand those ideologies. In particular, why have certain ideologies been adopted? We need to do this in the belief that understanding the reasons for others' positions is as important as having good defences for our own (Bonnett, 2001). Addressing this process aspect of the difficulty of different ontological and epistemological positions is as important as working on the content. In fact, if we only considered one or the other, we wouldn't properly be developing critical perspectives on health.

The Difficulty of the Impact of Professional Beliefs and Values on Our Conceptions of Health: Content and Process

My argument here is that professional education and training heavily but subtly inculcates within us a particular set of professional beliefs and values about the nature of 'health'. In general, professionals incline towards objectivist, positivist conceptions of health.

The *content* challenge within this difficulty is to try and identify the beliefs and values held by professionals about the nature of 'health' and to assess the worth of these. The *process* challenge is partly to recognise the existence of particular beliefs and values, especially given my argument that the way in which these are imparted to us is hidden and full of nuance. It is also about trying to understand why it is that, as professionals, we hold the beliefs and values that we do about the nature of health.

The Difficulty of Attempting to Understand Academic Disciplinary Discourses Related to Health: Content and Process

If the idea of 'health' is subject to a range of treatments by different academic disciplines, then we need to familiarise ourselves with a variety of disciplinary discourses. We also need to be able to move easily between different disciplines and different interpretations.

The *content* challenge here involves the examination of particular disciplinary discourses with the purpose of trying to work out whether the assumptions that are being made and the argumentation being employed is justified. Ultimately, it's about assessing the worth of the particular discipline's putative contribution to understanding the idea of 'health'. The *process* challenge, on the other hand, is equally to examine the discourses. But this time it's with the purpose of trying to understand why the discipline concerned is actually taking a particular direction, together with how (and why) its moves might resemble, or fail to resemble, moves and argumentation we might be familiar with from other disciplines. Is there a similarity? Why? If there is similarity (or difference), what can we learn from this to help future approaches to this or other disciplines?

For example, I might consider a discourse from psychology – say one that was about considering the place of self-efficacy in HIV prevention (i.e., the role of the individual in determining their own capacity to minimise the risk of infection by HIV) (Maibach and Murphy, 1995). I might recognise the concern within this discourse to try and establish 'self-efficacy' as something that was quantifiable and could therefore be measured. This might in turn match up with my previous familiarity with the discipline of epidemiology and its concern with quantifiability and measurement. Then I might consider why psychology, at least in this particular discourse, resembles the discourse of epidemiology. What might this tell me about the purpose and direction of psychology, given that I'm approaching it with little experience of how it works (but with some experience of the workings of epidemiology)? In this way, examination of *process* starts to tell us quite a lot about how disciplines operate, about the similarities and differences between them and in turn our capacity for interdisciplinary understanding is increased.

Thinking Point

Do you agree with the distinctions that I've drawn between *content* and *process* in relation to the central difficulties of health studies that I've identified so far? Are the distinctions clear enough, or is the division between content and process blurred in some way? If it is, what might this tell us about the nature of health studies, its difficulties and how we might try to understand and deal with them?

What Needs to be Done to Start Dealing with the Component Difficulties of 'The Difficulty of Health Studies'?

I want to argue now that careful thinking about the central components of 'the difficulty of health studies', along with their content and process elements, leads to recognition that we need to engage with them intellectually in two kinds of ways if we are to address them properly. (I'm using the term 'intellectual' in a general sense at the moment to signify the use and development of our capacity to acquire knowledge and to reason so that in some way we can understand our world, or part of that world, better.)

▸ These two ways are *critical analysis;*
▸ And *critical reflection.*

I'll start now to call both of these ways processes. I'm using the term as I did before; these are actions or operations we need to undertake in order to understand problems more fully. It's important to realise, however, that proper application of the processes of critical analysis and critical reflection ought to benefit not only the *process* difficulties I've identified but also the *content* ones.

It's pretty certain that you will have come across the terms 'critical analysis' and 'critical reflection' before. My guess is that it might also well be the case that in your studies at some point, you've been encouraged to develop your 'skills of critical analysis and critical reflection'. Within your academic experience, you will probably have talked with lecturers and tutors about both of these things. It makes sense, then, to ask a couple of questions aimed at working out whether your own understanding of 'critical analysis' and 'critical reflection' in the context of health studies marries with my own.

Thinking Point

Before considering my own response to questions about the nature of critical analysis and critical reflection, think about your own. What do you currently understand by the terms 'critical analysis' and 'critical reflection'? On the basis of your current understanding of what the terms involve, and on your reaction to the argument I've set out for the difficulty in studying health, why might they be important for the health studies student?

The Need for Critical Analysis

I understand 'critical analysis' as:

▸ An intellectual process that attempts to understand the meaning and nature of something (an idea, a concept, a theory, a 'real world' phenomenon) by examining it in detail (Tate, 2004).

Analysis of something involves breaking it down into its constituent parts and examining each part carefully so that finally we have a fuller picture of the thing itself (Marshall and Rowland, 1998: 88). Although we are involved with conceptual and theoretical analysis, it is worth reflecting for a moment on the *scientific* process of analysis. Indeed, some dictionaries foreground the idea of scientific analysis within their general definitions of the word 'analysis':

To separate (a substance etc.) into its parts in order to identify it or study its structure. (Oxford University Press, 1983: 20)

A pharmacist, for example, might be asked to examine an unidentified substance. To begin with, she would examine the substance macroscopically (that is to say, just by looking at it with the naked eye, perhaps performing tests to separate the substance out or to witness any readily visible changes in colour or structure). Doing these things might enable her to establish what the substance was. However, the results of this kind of examination and this testing may mean that she still cannot be sure about the nature of the substance. So she resorts to microscopic examination (looking at the substance through a microscope and possibly submitting it to testing and microscopy). In this way, she can identify the structure of the substance and so name the substance itself.

Now take the thing that we have been considering and discussing – the idea of 'health'. Although it's not nearly as readily confined as the unidentified substance in the pharmacy example, and a microscope isn't going to do us much good, we're actually trying to engage in very similar processes. We've been presented with 'health'. This is the 'substance', if you like, that we've been asked to examine. We might initially have felt a high degree of certainty that we knew what it was – the absence of disease, say. Then we started to examine this notion and realised it didn't quite fit in with other things we seemed to recognise about health. For example, someone could perfectly sensibly regard himself as healthy even though he might be suffering from chronic physical disease. Then we started to engage in what could be regarded as our own equivalent of microscopic examination. We began to look at what it was that provided the structure to the complex 'substance' we now realised that we were dealing with. We began to build up a picture of the 'substance' being structured by professional ideologies, beliefs and values; and also by particular academic perspectives. This is pretty much the point we're at now.

I don't want to stretch the comparison between the pharmacy example and our own enterprise too far; there are obvious differences. My point is that the process of analysis is central in getting a fuller, more complete account of 'health', the thing we are attempting to study and which is perplexing us so much. What is key is that we are engaged in *critical* analysis; an evaluative process through which we 'identify, uncover and sometimes counter assertions and assumptions' (Bonnett, 2001: 105). In this way, our analysis becomes a matter of saying not only, for example, that the idea of 'health' is subject to interpretation; but also of examining *why* we might believe this, what alternative positions there might be and why we might hold such positions.

So one essential difference between the scientific (pharmacy) example of analysis and our own kind of analytical enquiry is this. The pharmacist, having broken down the unidentified substance into its component parts and therefore worked out what it actually is, might be happy to leave things there. This is paracetamol, say, or glycerol. There is not necessarily a reason to move beyond 'what?' questions to 'why?' ones. Sometimes, of course, this may be required. (Say she was involved in a police investigation and was speculating about why a drug dealer was using crushed paracetamol to resemble heroin to his unsuspecting punters.) Frequently, though, working out what something actually is constitutes the end-product of analysis in the physical sciences. For us however, the task of analysis – critical analysis – *essentially* involves asking 'why?' questions, of building up argument and counter-argument (Bonnett, 2001: 103). These kinds of questions are fundamental, given the contested and disputed nature of much of the territory of health studies. Nothing can be taken for granted.

Critical analysis is primarily a cognitive process (Tate, 2004). It involves a certain kind of thinking that it's possible broadly to characterise as being directed towards reasoning, the justification of particular positions or assumptions and argumentation (Marshall and Rowland, 1998). This in turn implies that attempting critical analysis also involves trying to achieve a degree of objectivity in your thinking, of trying to remove yourself from the context and allowing the argumentation you've developed to speak for itself. Of course, I don't mean to suggest that we should avoid feeling strongly (even passionately!) about the positions we are trying to justify or about the argument we are trying to develop. I might believe, for example, that an 'absence of disease' view of health is completely inadequate because it fails to take seriously notions such as social and emotional well-being. I might think that the person who doesn't take such things seriously is shallow-thinking and wrong-headed. But if this were all I thought, then I wouldn't be engaging in critical analysis. For my position to become critically analytic, I need to recognise the other person's position and to understand why they hold it. I need to work out where and why it harbours weaknesses. I need to compare it with my own. I need to use the theoretical and empirical evidence available to me in order to establish the strengths of my position over my opponent's, as well as the truths that more than likely lie somewhere within what they are saying. I need to do all these things because there is a requirement to advance in our understanding of the conceptually and practically problematic field of health.

But while engaging in critical analysis is a *necessary* condition for deeper understanding of 'the difficulty of health studies', it isn't a *sufficient* one. It can't be, given how I've mapped and described the difficulty. The kinds of problems we face are two-fold:

▸ Trying to make sense of competing conceptual, theoretical and empirical understandings;
▸ Attempting to work out what ideologies, beliefs and values underpin these understandings.

Critical analysis will certainly help with the first kind of problem. To some extent it will also help with the second. But it won't tell the whole story, simply because *we ourselves possess health-related beliefs and values*. We need to recognise the values and beliefs that we hold, and we need to try and work out why we hold them. Doing so requires critical *reflection*, as well as critical analysis, to play a fundamental part in understanding 'the difficulty of health studies'.

The Need for Critical Reflection

What is critical reflection? My view is that at its heart:

> It is thinking about your own thinking and about your own experiences in a way that enables you to learn from these deliberations. (Marshall and Rowland, 1998: 8)

The implication of this idea of learning from reflecting on your thinking and on your experiences is that in some way it will offer you the opportunity to *change* how you think and what you do.

The opportunity that processes of critical reflection appear to allow for change and development, particularly in the context of professional training, work and continuing development have made it an important policy and education imperative for health care professional work particularly. (See, for example, Dietitians' Board, 2000; General Medical Council, 1993; United Kingdom Central Council for Nursing, Midwifery and Health Visiting, 1986.) Policy and education imperative has been accompanied by an expanding theoretical literature, as well as work that aims to connect the theory of critical reflection and reflective practice (very often the terms are used synonymously) to how they can be implemented in training and work contexts. (See, for example, Burns and Bulman, 2000; Tate and Sills, 2004; Rolfe, Freshwater and Jasper, 2001.)

Thinking Point

If you are able, have a look again at your own profession's guidance or requirements with regard to the development of reflective practice; and the reflective capacity of its members or members-in-training. What requirements is your profession making of you?

If you are currently undertaking an academic programme or course, have a look at the course/programme learning outcomes

Thinking Point *continued*

that might relate to critical reflection and reflective practice. (There should be at least some, certainly if you are studying in the United Kingdom, as the ideas are prominent in subject benchmarking statements from the Quality Assurance Agency for Higher Education and other relevant bodies. What academic expectations are you being presented with? How are you fulfilling these (or how are you planning to fulfil them)? What support are you getting to help you fulfil these expectations?

Reviewing the range of theoretical, policy and practice literature related to critical reflection and reflective practice in health care would take up several volumes by itself. My own discussion must be heavily circumscribed. But there are important questions that I want to raise at this point. There is a set of questions related to the demand being placed on you – as a student or as a practitioner – with regard to the development of critical reflective capacity. They are essentially the kinds of questions posed in the 'Thinking Point' above. I have asked them with a particular motivation, based on certain understandings of the place of critical reflection in professional training and academic education. My understanding of the potential problematic of critical reflection in the development of health care professionals is this:

▶ It may be the case that students or practitioners are unclear of the demands made by professions, and the commitment required of the professions' members, to the idea and ideal of critical reflection and reflective practice (Fade, 2004).
▶ There is sometimes a feeling that reflection – thinking about what you've experienced and done and changing your practice in the light of such thought – is 'Easy peasy', or, 'We do it anyway, we don't need to think about it' (Jones, 2004).
▶ Levels of capacity for learning and teaching in this area vary between academics – even academics teaching and lecturing on vocational training programmes and courses (Fade, 2004; Young, 2004).

Given these things, both learners and teachers alike might one way or another be grappling with the idea of critical reflection and reflective practice: what it actually is; what demands it makes of individuals; ways of encouraging and assessing it, among other things. The questions in the 'Thinking Point' above are aimed at encouraging your own thought about the demands placed on you by the idea of critical reflection. You could also perhaps use them to stimulate conversations between yourself, your peers and your teachers about the requirements of critical reflection in the context of 'the difficulty of health studies'.

There are two further questions about the idea of critical reflection that I want to ask now:

▸ Why is the idea of critical reflection so prominent in health care education policy and practice?
▸ Why exactly is critical reflection important for tackling 'the difficulty of health studies' as I've described and discussed it?

The two questions are in fact closely connected. Responses to both will contribute to developing an agenda for dealing with 'the difficulty of health studies'.

Why has Critical Reflection Become so Important?

Commentators point to a number of reasons for the 'rise' of critical reflection. There is a belief that the increasingly complex nature of our society demands much greater complexity in professionals' responses to meeting the needs – including the need of 'health' – within the public they 'profess' (Koehn, 1994) to serve. Professionals can no longer rely on a single, discrete body of knowledge to last them through 30–40 years or more of their working lives (Powell, 1999). They need to be able to deal with evermore difficult situations, to dwell for longer and longer periods in what Schön (1987: 3) calls 'the swampy lowlands of professional practice.' Part of their capacity to do this depends on their ability to learn from their experiences – in other words, to reflect (Tate, 2004).

Broader social changes are also mirrored in the shifting context of health care (and health care-related education). Professionals are encouraged to see individuals as people rather than as 'bits to be fixed' – 'broken legs' or 'stomach ulcers' or whatever (Cribb and Duncan, 2002). There is a dominating policy requirement for our work with patients, newly reconstituted as people, so to speak, to be 'effective' and to be based on 'evidence' (White, 2004). This is at least partly because these 'new' people are no longer passive, broken bits – they have turned into active and challenging consumers (Cooter, 2000).

In turn, this policy requirement has led to a much-increased emphasis in recent years on health care professionals developing effective clinical decision making supported by robust clinical reasoning. It's suggested that the demands made by these processes can at least in part be met by encouraging capacity for critical reflection (White, 2004).

So it's possible to argue that the idea and practice of clinical reflection in health care has emerged so strongly because:

▸ Health care professionals need to deal with highly complex situations;
▸ Health care consumers expect professionals to be able to do so.

If these reasons for the importance of critical reflection in health care practice sound familiar, I hope that it's at least partly because they bear strong resemblance to some of the reasons I've so far discussed for 'the difficulty of health studies'. In Chapter 2, I thought about societal complexity, the emergence of professions and growing critiques of professional power. I did this to build my case for seeing professional values and beliefs related to health as strong, pervasive and very hard to change. Now we see critical reflection (a potential tool for dealing with difficulties related to the study of health) itself emerging as a result of the need health care professionals have to meet the requirements of an evermore complex and demanding society. In Chapter 3, I focused specifically on the shifting context of health care and health care-related education, partly to demonstrate the difficulty for the person studying health in getting a purchase on disciplinary and interdisciplinary thinking. Now critical reflection is seen, too, as a way of supporting processes such as clinical reasoning and clinical decision making, required partly as a result of society's strident demands for effective services. The requirement for clinical reasoning can also be seen as moving practitioners towards ways of working out how to function appropriately in constantly altering contexts, of both practice and education for practice (White, 2004).

While I want to point to a resemblance between my arguments for 'the difficulty of health studies' and the emergence of critical reflection as a way of coping with problems in health care, I don't want to make too much of it. Apart from anything else, it would seem too neat! Critical reflection as an idea, as a concept and as practice is difficult. But thinking more about its nature might help us to work out exactly why it's important in tackling the problems of health studies. It might also help to align the difficulties we've been discussing so far with the broader problems of professional education and practice that critical reflection is seen as central in helping to clarify and resolve.

Academics and those involved in professional education have traditionally viewed the development of learning as being based on processes of cognition that are about reasoning, along with argumentation and its justification. These things encourage learners to place themselves in positions of objective scrutiny. They are the kinds of cognitive processes that I associated earlier with critical analysis. If they have sounded familiar to you, it is possibly because they have dominated higher and professional education for many years. But for the reasons I've just discussed, the difficult and constantly changing contexts of what we might call late modern society (Ball, 2003) have rendered education and professional training that focuses solely on processes of objective scrutiny as inadequate. With this realisation, educational theorists began to develop strong and coherent accounts of learning that suggest it is an incomplete process unless the *whole person* is involved (Claxton, 1988). Not many of us would probably wish to describe ourselves as wholly rational. We would presumably want to talk about ourselves as people who pursue rationality some of the time, but who also act in ways that sometimes are not particularly rational and who experience feelings that frequently move us to believe and behave in certain non-rational ways. So if we want to understand ourselves properly, if we want to engage as a whole person in learning, we need to move beyond objectivity and rationality. We need to recognise and attend to our feelings and emotions – what Honey and Mumford (1986) refer to as our *affective domain*. Objective reasoning and rational justification is certainly important, but it can't help us to make complete sense of what we encounter and have to deal with – our experiences – simply because of who we are as people. Critical reflection centrally involves exploration of *feelings* as an important part of our experiences, as well as the thoughts and actions that also helped form particular experience (Boud, Keogh and Walker, 1985).

Theorists have developed a number of different models of reflective learning. The one that I'm presenting here is really no more than my personal choice – it makes sense to me as a representation of what might happen within the process of critical reflection. It's important, however, to emphasise that what theorists have done is simply to construct *models* – representations of reality and not reality itself. In the same way that the map of the London Underground is a model of the

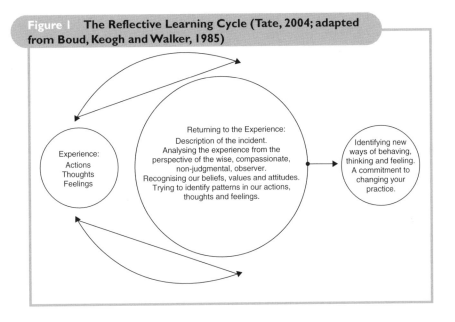

Figure 1   The Reflective Learning Cycle (Tate, 2004; adapted from Boud, Keogh and Walker, 1985)

Experience:
Actions
Thoughts
Feelings

Returning to the Experience:
Description of the incident.
Analysing the experience from the
perspective of the wise, compassionate,
non-judgmental, observer.
Recognising our beliefs, values and attitudes.
Trying to identify patterns in our actions,
thoughts and feelings.

Identifying new
ways of behaving,
thinking and feeling.
A commitment to
changing your
practice.

Tube (thousands of curves straightened out, stations placed on it in ways that help us get where we want to go), what I've presented is a *model of reflection*. The actual real-life Tube has complexities that it wouldn't be helpful to try and present on the map (even if that was possible). This (and other models of reflective learning) can't completely express the complexities of the process.

In particular, what I've presented (Figure 1) is a model of a certain kind of reflective learning – what Schön (1987) would call 'reflection *on* action'. This is reflection sometime after a particular experience. It contrasts with his idea of 'reflection *in* action'. In this latter way of reflecting, an individual engages in the reflective process while they are actually in a particular experience, doing so in a way that we can probably best describe as intuitive. Reflection *in* action is a characteristic of the expert – rather than the novice – practitioner (Benner, 1984).

My assumption now is that you as the reader of this book, and myself as the author, are both partly engaged in the process of reflection *on* action. My hope is that in part what this book is doing is to encourage you to reflect at a distance on your cumulative experience of the idea of health and health-related practices. I hope that it is encouraging you both through processes of rationality and objectivity, as well as processes that stimulate examination of thoughts and feelings, to use your past experiences to reconstruct, or perhaps to reconfirm, your understanding of health.

Broadly, then, if we are engaged in this kind of project of reflection *on* action, the model that I've presented suggests we need to go through two sorts of stages in order to reflect on action, on our experience.

▸ We need to begin by describing the experience, in a way that not only depicts what took place (actions) but also how we thought and felt about it.

▸ Then we need to reflect on it 'with the intention of coming to new understandings' (Tate, 2004:11).

I'll consider in more detail how this reflection might take place in Chapter 6. In a general sense, though, what is important at this second stage is that we approach reflection, as far as possible, not with the intention of giving ourselves a hard time over what has happened but instead with the purpose of constructing and using our reflections positively. Tate (2004: 13) talks of the need for us to attempt taking on the role of a 'wise, compassionate, non-judgmental observer of our own experience.'

Why is this focus on affection – on taking account of our feelings and emotions as well as of our 'rational self' – so important in addressing 'the difficulty of health studies'? The answer lies partly in thinking again about the theory underpinning the idea of critical reflection. If we fail to take account of domains beyond the rational, if we ignore affection, then we are neglecting to do justice to ourselves as learners who are not simply learners but people as well. The answer also lies in the nature of 'the difficulty of health studies' itself. In the 'process' and 'content' analysis of the difficulty that I undertook earlier, I placed a significant emphasis on the need to recognise the ideologies surrounding theoretical constructions of health. I also emphasised the need to relate these ideologies to the beliefs and values that we possess by virtue of our personal, and particularly our professional, backgrounds. My assertion is that because we are talking of ourselves as people here – influenced as well as influencing, subjects as well as (probably more than) independent rationalists – we can only properly consider the place of values and beliefs in understandings of health if we carefully examine our feelings and emotions.

Thinking Point

Do you agree with my assertion that examination of feelings and emotions can help proper consideration of the foundations and nature of our beliefs and values and the relationship between these things and how we think about 'health'? If you agree, why? If you don't, why not?

If you do agree with me, what difficulties might you face in such examination? How would you overcome them?

What is the Relationship between Critical Analysis and Critical Reflection?

I want to emphasise that critical analysis and critical reflection are not processes that are divorced from each other. If we are to properly understand 'the difficulty of health studies', we need to engage in both. This is essential because dealing with the difficulty involves:

▸ Tackling theoretical and empirical argument (in which critical *analysis* becomes central) and;
▸ Understanding values and beliefs (where critical *reflection* is fundamental).

Perhaps, though, you are still concerned that in some way the two processes are disconnected and that because of this, it will be much harder to tackle the problems that we face. After all, one is about fostering objectivity, while the other is what some people might call 'touchy-feely'.

My inclination is to follow Tate (2004) and regard critical analysis and critical reflection as the same kind of process, but operating within different paradigms. Both involve cognition (thinking). Whether we are attempting rationally to justify or attack assumptions, or to consider our feelings about a particular experience, we are obviously required to think. But whereas critical analysis demands that we adopt the position of the detached, rational objectivist, critical reflection urges us to involve ourselves in the situation we are experiencing. So we can see them as similar processes, but operating according to different sorts of world view. Critical reflection belongs to what Schön (1987) calls the 'professional artistry' model, while critical analysis belongs to 'technical-rational'. They are two sides of the same coin. If we are conscientious professionals, we cannot accept a commitment to one without also being similarly committed to the other.

Shaping a Response to 'The Difficulty of Health Studies'

I've argued that responding to 'the difficulty of health studies' requires us to engage in processes of both critical analysis and critical reflection. So part of a response to the difficulty must be about developing skills in relation to each of the processes, mindful of the need to address the components of the difficulty that we've identified. Part II of this book – Chapters 5 and 6 – considers the processes and how they might be developed.

In Chapter 5, I focus on the process of critical analysis. How can evidence and argument in relation to the idea of 'health', which claims to be rational, be examined? How can we move towards properly justified argument? How is it possible to deconstruct and detect weaknesses in the argumentation of others?

In Chapter 6, I move to thinking about the process of critical reflection in relation to 'the difficulty of health studies'. How might we be able to examine situations and experiences that contribute to our idea of 'health' and the problems associated with its study? How can we deal with issues that this might raise for us in terms of our professional training and development, and our academic education?

Equipped, I hope, with an understanding of the processes and skills required for tackling problems in the study of health, I want then to move to thinking about particular difficulties and the demands that they appear to make. The way that I intend to do this is to examine a small number of different disciplinary discourses related to the idea of 'health' and 'the difficulty of health studies'. What I want to emphasise here is that my primary intention is not to try and clarify exactly the kind of contribution that a particular discipline can make to thinking about and studying 'health'. This is something that other texts (e.g., Naidoo and Wills, 2001) have as their express purpose.

My own intention in this book is to examine the discourses of the disciplines I've chosen and to apply the processes and skills I've associated with the development of genuinely critical perspectives (critical analysis and critical reflection) to *some* of the understandings offered by these disciplines. In this way, my aim is to show the worth (or otherwise) of what purport to be critical perspectives on health and on 'the difficulty of health studies'. The end stage of all this should be the identification of problems and possibilities within a range of discourses, which might in turn move us towards responding to the component problems I've identified, and to the overall difficulty. There may be no definitive answers – or you may disagree with the responses I've come up with – but what I hope is that the process will have been one of genuine critical engagement.

The disciplinary discourses related to health that I have chosen to examine are these. In Chapter 7, I want to consider some philosophical discourses on health and the assumptions and arguments they seem to be making about the *nature* of health – the ontological and epistemological foundations of our understanding of the concept. In Chapter 8, I will use the values-related discourses of ethics to establish their worth in relation to developing understanding around ideas of the *value* of 'health', and health-related practices. Following this, in Chapter 9, I consider sociological discourses, which seem to me to exemplify debates about where power and control over health is located and views about how health is '*produced*'. Finally, in Chapter 10, I try and draw lessons from my examination of these discourses and attempt to establish how it might be possible to continue developing critical perspectives on health.

There is of course a much broader range of disciplines that are likely to be useful in developing critical perspectives on health. I have touched on some of these already-history and psychology, for example. In fact, other disciplines such as these contribute to debates within the disciplinary discourses I have chosen to examine. This perhaps emphasises the developing interdisciplinary nature of studies related to health. But I also hope that this book will stimulate you to go on and examine this broader range of health-related disciplines in more detail.

Biomedicine and Critical Perspectives on Health

One of the criticisms that could be levelled at this plan for developing a response to the difficulties that have been identified in studying health is that it fundamentally neglects biomedicine. (In talking about 'biomedicine', I mean the cluster of disciplines and sub-disciplines that contribute to medical practice, as well as medicine itself. These would include biology, anatomy, physiology, pathology and epidemiology.)

It's quite possible that someone could make the following argument against the plan I'm proposing:

> *You've discussed at some length the nature of argumentation – normative, analytic and so on – and warned us to beware of unjustified changes in styles of argumentation. Remember your argument from Psychology in Chapter Three? You asserted that the authors of the Health Action Model had switched their argument from analytic to normative. They had moved – without being explicit that they'd done so – from an argument that was basically explanatory to one in which norms and standards had already been assumed prior to argument; in this case that health behaviour change was a worthwhile activity. But now you're doing exactly the same thing, except this time on a book-wide scale!*
>
> *By excluding the medical sciences from your examinations of disciplinary discourse, you are assuming (without telling us) a normative position. The position is this. You believe that in order to move towards an understanding of the difficulty in studying health, part of what we need to do is to consider critically discourses on health from philosophy, sociology and so on. These discourses propose themselves as offering 'critical perspectives' on the field that we are studying. Your plan is to critically assess, as it were, these so-called critical perspectives. But in removing the medical sciences from the debate, you are adopting a normative position. You are implying (without actually saying) that medical sciences, by virtue of their concern with quantifiability, their orientation towards viewing health as a fixed state – the absence of disease – do not and cannot adopt critical perspectives on health Surely medicine is worth more than this blithe rejection.*

This is a reasonable argument and I need to defend myself against it. In the first place, I'm happy to acknowledge that in at least some quarters of the medical sciences, positions on the issues that I have been discussing are much more reflexive than the fixed state my imagined opponent assumes that I believe in. As Benton (1991: 23) reminds us, positions in the biological and medical sciences are often both fluid and critically analytic, particularly in areas such as sociobiology. Second, biomedicine hasn't in fact been absent from my arguments so far, nor will it be from the disciplinary perspectives I will be examining. If anything, quite the reverse is the case.

Up to this point, what I've earlier called 'the shadow of biomedicine' has often loomed over my arguments. It will continue to do so right the way through the rest of the text. This has to be the case because biomedicine is one of the central forces (probably the most central force) driving argument and debate in the field of health studies. I agree that I am not examining discourses from biomedicine itself. But what I am doing is considering discourses that, one way or another, have all been profoundly influenced by biomedicine. So the medical sciences have a central place in our discussions. It really couldn't be otherwise.

Turning Point?

At the beginning of this chapter, I asked you to review what you'd read so far and list what occurred to you as the key issues and questions related to 'the difficulty of health studies'. Now you've finished reading the chapter, I hope that you're in a position to confirm your understanding of the issues is the same as mine, or to recognise any differences.

Whether or not there are differences between us over key issues and questions, it could still be the case that you disagree with the plan I've put forward for tackling difficulties. In particular:

▸ Am I right in bringing to the foreground the disciplinary discourses that I do?

▸ Am I right in regarding the medical sciences as a pervasive shadow over the disciplines, a 'theme' if you like (and possibly not a very positive one) rather than something very much in the foreground of the picture?

If you agree with the plan that I've set out, consider your reasons for doing so and justify them. If you disagree, consider and justify your reasons also. In addition, set out your own alternative plan for tacking 'the difficulty of health studies' and justify this.

What's gone on in this chapter?

I've developed a sense of the importance of both critical analysis and critical reflection as processes that will help us understand better 'the difficulty of health studies'. We need critical *analysis* in order to tackle the theoretical and empirical argument that makes up much of the territory of health studies. We need critical *reflection* in order to understand and deal with the values and beliefs that underlie the territory. These processes, and their related skills, need to be applied to a small number of academic disciplinary discourses on 'health', which purport to tell us something useful about the concept. So the agenda for the rest of the book has been set out.

Part II
Developing Critical
Perspectives

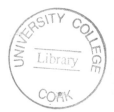

Health Studies and Critical Analysis

What is this chapter going to do?

This chapter considers in more detail the relationship between health studies and critical analysis, one of the process elements I've argued is necessary for tackling difficulties within the field. I identify ways in which we can go about critically analysing argument, relate these to the kinds of arguments that we are likely to find in the health studies field and move towards a 'set of procedures' for the examination of health-related argument.

Critical Analysis, Argument and Health

I've argued that the processes of critical analysis and critical reflection are essential in dealing with 'the difficulty of health studies'. If we are serious in our study of health, then we need to develop our understanding and skills in relation to both processes. In this chapter, I consider the process of critical analysis.

Much of the Chapter's focus relates to the critical analysis of written argument. The reason for this focus is simple. Written argument and argumentation are central to the development of positions in the field of health studies and to the advancement, justification and defence of those positions. So critical analysis, the cognitive process of reasoning and the justification of particular positions or assumptions must essentially be about the careful examination of argument. Health studies students need to develop the capacity to ponder, examine and critically analyse the written argument of those who claim to have discovered something about 'health', or health care-related practices.

The Chapter has three main aspects:

▸ I want to develop my justification for seeing critical analysis as central to unravelling the problems involved in studying health. Critical analysis is a demanding intellectual process so we need to be clear that it's worthwhile;

▸ I also want to examine ways in which we might understand the process of argument better and so develop our capacity to engage in critically analytic ways with the arguments that fill the field of health studies;

▸ I want in addition to consider an issue that seems to perplex both learners and teachers in the field, as well as in other academic arenas. This is the issue of whether the capacity for critical analysis is innate (a bit like musical ability, perhaps) or whether it can be learnt (in the same way that we are all capable of learning a broad range of other kinds of skills). This is a central issue for those involved in learning and teaching in health studies, as in other areas.

Critical analysis of argument, of understanding how and why someone has adopted the position that they have and evaluating its worth and strength, is an illuminating and rewarding academic process. As Bonnett puts it:

> The ability to engage in argument is what makes learning exciting. (Bonnett, 2001: 1)

But engaging in the critical analysis of others' arguments is not necessarily the end in itself. If we do engage ourselves in this way, what should ultimately happen is that we begin to develop positions of our own. If we see difficulties in someone else's perspective, we start to counter-argue: 'This can't be the case and if that's so, then maybe *this* is a more reasonable position instead.' In turn, we may come across another position that causes us further to refine the one we thought reasonable. So analysis of argument and counter-argument leads us to our own position. This may not be burning with novelty and originality – how many of us are able to come up with regular supplies of earth-shattering ideas? – but it will be *distinctive* because it is the sound product of careful thought and the result of our active engagement with the world of ideas.

Why are Argument and its Critical Analysis Important in Health Studies?

The development, understanding and critique of reasoning and argument are essential to all academic disciplines and fields of study (Bonnett, 2001; Fairbairn and Winch, 1998). These things are (or should be) the features of academic activity that mark it out as a distinctive and fundamental form of human enquiry. But there are three particular reasons why argument is so important in the field of health studies. These reasons stem from 'the difficulty of health studies' itself.

Health is Contested – We can Assume Nothing about It

First, much of our discussion so far has centred round the idea of 'health' as a contested concept and consequently the view that has emerged of health studies is as a contested field. 'Health' is contested in ontological and epistemological terms; and this contest is underpinned and fed by ideological and values-related disputes. Contest and dispute creates argument; argument creates contest and dispute. Gallie (1956: 167) talks of the potential for contest in relation to 'any concept of common sense or of the natural sciences', but argues for the existence of especially virulent contest in those areas where assumptions can't be made about the nature of the concept concerned. I hope my discussions so far have confirmed that we can *assume* nothing about the nature of health (and thus of related concepts and practices). So if we are to advance in our understanding, we need to move from simple (and disputable) assumption of positions to their *justification* – or reasoned rejection of justifications that have been offered. This is the territory of argument and its analysis.

Understanding Health Requires us to Analyse Multiple Perspectives

Second, I've argued for the view that a single disciplinary perspective just wouldn't be enough to capture or attempt to make sense of the complexity of the concept of health. If this is so, then our encounter with a variety of different disciplinary beliefs, assumptions and values will require us to formulate and defend, or alternatively to critique, a range of different positions emerging from a number of different disciplines. This is difficult, not least because as I discussed in Chapter 3 separate disciplines possess their 'own' language. They may also operate according to certain general disciplinary *heuristics*-what might be described as 'rule of thumb' procedures that set the person enquiring broadly in the direction of a correct response (in the discipline's terms) to the problem with which they have been presented (Powell, 1999: 22). For example, sociologists might use a particular range of qualitative research methods with a given community to explore that community's idea of 'health'. Philosophers, on the other hand, may confine themselves to examining particular kinds of wholly theoretical argument to develop an understanding of the concept. They may go nowhere near people or communities! (And in the discipline's terms, this wouldn't be a problem.)

The fact that separate disciplines operate with different sets of heuristics doesn't mean that one set, and the outcomes it leads to, should be regarded as somehow more preferable or 'better' than another is. Whichever discipline careful and thoughtful contributions to the concept of health and the field of health studies come from, and whatever particular set of heuristics have underpinned the contribution, it's likely to be of help to us. What it does mean, though, is that we have to be very careful in analysing the stages which the person whose argument we are considering, whatever their 'primary' discipline, went through in order to reach their conclusions.

My own view is that in thinking about the nature of argument, it's possible to establish what we might call a set of heuristics for the examination of positions in the field of health studies. With some circumscriptions and limitations, this kind of device might help give us confidence that although we are working in a field, and encountering a range of disciplines, we are doing so in a robust and thoughtful way. I'll come back to the idea of a set of heuristics for analysing health studies-related arguments later in the chapter.

Thinking Point

What are the *heuristics* – the 'guiding rules of thumb' – of the academic discipline with which you have most affinity? To what extent do you think they contribute towards the discipline's effective exploration of the territory encompassed by health studies? To what extent do the heuristics themselves make effective exploration of the territory more difficult?

We 'Apply' the Arguments of Health Studies – So we Need to Be as Sure of Them as Possible

My third point in support of the view that argument and its analysis are centrally important in the field of health studies relates to the nature of the field itself and its application. While health studies is a field of academic study, it is what can be called an 'applied' field. When we analyse and discuss the nature of health, what it might mean and how it might be represented, we are often doing so with a particular purpose. Our intention is very often to try and understand how things could be better arranged or conducted in the real world of practice. So there is the distinct possibility that our academic work can (arguably should) be applied to such contexts. If I ask the question, 'What is health?' and come to the conclusion that its meaning depends on interpretation and could be understood as, for example, 'the foundations for achievement', then this will have practical implications. It will mean something in terms of the way I perceive my professional role, and how I envisage and undertake my professional practice. In turn, this will result in practice and professional implications for the people who manage and direct me. It will mean, for example, that I might encourage someone to reject the medication for depression that he's been prescribed because after long conversations we have agreed that it is inhibiting his emotional and psychological state. It is preventing the development of his 'foundations'. This direction will have important implications not just for the person I am trying to help, but also for myself as the practitioner, as well as for my managers.

The conversion of abstract discussion into talk with purpose and meaning in the real world has important consequences. While I would argue that it's quite reasonable to regard abstract and conceptual talk as useful, practical relevance gives argument an essential added edge. We are no longer in the realms of the potentially ethereal. Instead, the results of our argument will affect people in real, everyday ways. Quite conceivably, our argument will ultimately make a difference between peoples' lives being on the one hand simply tolerable, and on the other positively worth living. It might possibly make the difference between good and bad lives, or even between life and death.

This suggestion is not as absurd as it might at first sound. If, for example, I'm convinced by an argument suggesting that health and human freedom are intimately connected, this will make it much easier for me to justify my view that life which is not 'free', for whatever reason, is not worth living (a life crippled by chronic degenerative disease, say). Alternatively, it might make it easier for someone to feel able to defend the view that lives they themselves construct as 'free, worthwhile and useful' are worth preserving and enhancing; and other lives (again according to their own constructions) are not. It is no accident that particular views of the nature of health, of the kinds of lives that need to be built or discouraged or even stopped – arguments of eugenics, in other words – have lain at the heart of totalitarian regimes such as Nazi Germany. And regimes such as Nazism have been moved to the most dreadful experiments and actions in the cause of creating and perpetuating what they have advocated as good (healthy) lives (Burleigh, 2001; Wörner, 2000).

If arguments about 'health' can be applied to our everyday lives (as I think they can and should be) it follows that our analysis of such arguments needs to be particularly robust. This is the case because of where both good and bad arguments have the potential to lead; that is to say, directly to individual lives and circumstances. But it is also the case because, if we are conscientious professionals, we need to be certain that our 'professions' (our declarations of help) (Koehn, 1994) to clients or patients who seek the good that we offer ('health', one way or another) are founded on solid ground. So our analysis of arguments related to health studies needs to have strength, and it needs to be conducted with care.

The Processes of Analysis and Argument: Differing Interpretations

I want to consider now two separate ways in which the process of argument itself has been explained and interpreted. In doing so, different positions on the nature of critical analysis, of how it can be learnt and taught, are uncovered:

▸ On the one hand there is the view of argument as a process that is hard to describe, or even that the best way of understanding it is as something intangible;

▸ On the other hand there is the idea that arguments possess structure, and this structure can be both identified and understood.

Thinking Point

Consider these two positions on the nature of the process of argument: the idea that argument is 'intangible'; and the idea that argument is something that can be identified, described and understood. If critical analysis is directed towards the appraisal and

Thinking Point *continued*

evaluation of argument, as I've suggested, as well as providing the foundation for developing our own distinctive arguments, what exactly *are* the implications of these two separate positions for health studies-related learning and teaching?

I'll begin with the idea that the process of argument is hard to grasp and rather intangible. This is an idea that Phyllis Creme and Mary Lea comment on in their book, 'Writing at University' (1997). It's important to recognise that one of the express purposes of Creme and Lea's book is to try and make explicit exactly how the kind of critical, analytic writing required of university students can be learnt and developed. But in order to move towards the position that such writing can be learnt, Creme and Lea work from one where the difficulties in doing so are acknowledged. They quote a university lecturer, one of the participants in their research on student writing:

> I can recognise a good piece of writing when I see it [the lecturer says]. I know when it is well structured and has a well-developed argument but it is difficult to say exactly what I am looking for, let alone describe a good argument more fully. (Creme and Lea, 1997: 37)

One of the findings of Creme and Lea's research is that this kind of view is relatively widespread among those who teach in higher education. There's a tendency to believe that the capacity to engage in critical analysis and to argue, at least as a writer, is something that you are 'either good at. ... or you are not' (Creme and Lea, 1997: 2).

This belief isn't unreasonable. Reflecting on my own experience, it's relatively easy to think of students who seem better able to analyse and argue than others. Those who are 'good' appear to be able to:

▸ Understand the assignment question that is being asked of them;
▸ Relate it to their theoretical encounters;
▸ Have the capacity to connect these to their own experience and to begin to develop analysis and argument that has relevance and direction.

Those who are less good seem to find it harder to do and demonstrate these things.

Yet from this highly anecdotal assessment of students' separate capacities for analysis and argumentation I move towards my preference for the other view of the process of arguments, the view that they do have structure, which can be identified and understood. As a lecturer I am able to start thinking (as I've just done) about the kinds of things going on in strong and less strong analysis and argument; understanding questions, developing relationships with theory and so on. This seems to me to be grounds for a reasonable belief that it's possible to work out what's happening in arguments: that their worth can be assessed; and so that critical analysis and argumentation can be *learnt and taught*.

Seeing it otherwise actually seems to me to be slightly disrespectful of individuals and their ability to engage with what are the nuts and bolts of academic life. It also appears quite disempowering. Believing that argument and analysis are important but essentially mysterious and therefore probably not teachable is a bit like someone saying, 'We want you to come and live in France. We realise that you can't speak French at the moment but we expect you to be able to do so by the time you arrive in the country. However, we don't really think you can manage this and we don't intend to offer you any language lessons or support to help you. But we still expect you to be able to speak French, and our reason for this is because **we** can.' I'm sure most people would see such a demand as neither particularly fair nor very empowering. And this is not so far off the situation where academics demand that students analyse critically and develop their own arguments, but expect them to be able to do so with little or no help. As Alastair Bonnett notes:

> Although arguing is vital for success in most disciplines the skills and culture of academic argument are rarely clearly introduced to students. (Bonnett, 2001: 2)

And if my assertion of the close relationship between argument and critical analysis is accepted – the latter as essential for both probing others' arguments and developing our own – then we might equally conclude that critical analysis suffers the same fate of rarely being clearly introduced.

Thinking Point

Consider your own experience so far as a health studies student. Have you engaged in active learning and teaching related to the development of skills of critical analysis? If so, how has this been done, who has been involved and what have been the outcomes for

Thinking Point *continued*

you, up to this point? If this hasn't happened in your case, what could you do now to support your learning in this area? It might be helpful to think about, list and investigate resources that could be available to you (e.g., study support unit, journal clubs, web-based learning, etc.). You could also frame a plan of action (e.g., 'talk to my tutor about how we could organise feedback on my assignments so that they focus more explicitly on what I need to do to develop my skills of critical analysis').

Understanding and Analysing Arguments

There is a range of potential reasons why the learning and teaching of argument and critical analysis is relatively neglected in higher education. Some of these relate to the nature of the processes themselves; it's true to say that understanding them better demands a lot of both teacher and learner. Some are connected to the nature of higher education itself, practice within the sector and the policy that influences it. This is perhaps especially so with regard to health care professional education in higher education. We might consider, for example, the policy changes I discussed earlier, which have tried to move health care professional curricula from a concern with peoples' 'broken bits' towards more holistic understandings. These attempts, as we've seen, have led to the focus in teaching being directed away from 'fact learning' to critical thinking and problem solving (Duncan, 2005). This broadening and deepening of health care professional education has also been embodied by the physical transfer of pre-qualification education in professions such as nursing into higher education (Eraut, 2002).

But like any major shift in policy and practice, this has not been without difficulties. For example, Eraut points to the lack of time and money available for research into the emerging 'new paradigm' of professional learning; and the slowness of transferring educational knowledge across disciplinary boundaries (Eraut, 2002: 1). These kinds of problems will certainly have affected the capacity of institutions and education professionals to engage with issues connected to the learning and teaching of the skills of critical analysis and argumentation (Stephenson, Higgs and Sugarman, 2001).

99

The Importance of Context in Argument and the Analysis of Argument

There are two reasons for my developing this argument for understanding why the learning and teaching of critical analysis and argumentation is relatively neglected in higher education:

▶ It sets my *specific argument* about the academic struggle with articulating and teaching the skills related to critical analysis and argument in a *broader context;*
▶ In doing so it demonstrates the importance of the fundamental stage of trying to *understand the context of an argument* in any analysis.

For arguments don't happen in vacuums. By definition, they involve exchange and debate (Oxford University Press, 1983: 30). According to Alastair Bonnett, academic argument is:

> A tool of learning and understanding. It is a form of intellectual **engagement**, a constructive intervention designed to contribute to a debate. As this implies, academic argument is a type of **exchange** based on sharing of knowledge, a pooling of facts and opinions. (Bonnett, 2001: 2)

As such, arguments take place in a context as well as forming part of that context. If we neglect context, we miss much about the argument itself. My own central argument in the first part of this book was for the existence of what I've called 'the difficulty of health studies'. But what sense would the argument have made if I'd neglected to describe and discuss its context? Say I hadn't talked about the dispute that exists over the nature and meaning of 'health'? Or I hadn't discussed the profound relationship between professional beliefs and values on the one hand and understandings of the idea of 'health' on the other? Or I hadn't examined the nature of disciplinary change and its relationship to altering conceptions of 'health'? I would want to claim that without these contextual explorations, my central argument – about 'the difficulty of health studies' – would have been dramatically weakened. In fact, I'm not sure that it could have been regarded as an argument at all.

Understanding of context is essential to the examination of any academic or academic-related argument. It applies whether we are trying to understand and critique the argument contained in a particular piece of policy, or whether we are considering a wholly theoretical argument.

Take the importance of context in understanding an argument within policy. An example of this is the first White Paper on health promotion and public health published by the 'New' Labour government – 'Saving Lives: Our Healthier Nation' (Secretary of State for Health, 1999). This document proposed target setting and action related to the prevention of morbidity and premature mortality in relation to a number of 'disease topics', including coronary heart disease (CHD) and stroke, and cancers. It was argued that action was required at three separate levels: the individual, the community and the government. Each had responsibilities and a part to play in reducing the toll of the preventable diseases considered by the White Paper.

'Saving Lives: Our Healthier Nation' is making a clear argument in favour of national health-related priorities and how it might be possible to deal with them. But we can only fully understand the nature and importance of the argument if we view it in context. We need to understand it as part of a response by a relatively wealthy economy (by global standards) to the so-called diseases of lifestyle and affluence (Priest and Speller, 1991) that exert considerable pressure on the health care resources of the rich western world. But we also need to recognise its focus, at least rhetorically, as being wider and more inclusive than the narrow individual lifestyle approach to disease prevention adopted by the Conservative government that preceded 'New' Labour. This was an approach widely and influentially criticised by health policy analysts (Benzeval, Judge and Whitehead, 1995; Francome and Marks, 1996). If we don't see the argument within the White Paper in the context of current and continuing health-related pressures and altered ways of seeing responsibilities for dealing with these, it is hard to see how a critically analytic perspective on its direction can be taken.

The need to examine context applies equally to arguments that might be seen as being mostly or wholly theoretical. At various points in my discussion so far, I've referred to the arguments of the philosopher W.B. Gallie (1956) in favour of the idea of 'essentially contested concepts'. The foundation for his argument is the idea that there are some concepts whose understanding seems subject to perpetual dispute. While some of Gallie's argument refers to examples from areas of practical concern such as democratic organisation and social justice, much of it appears to be highly abstract and theoretical – an argument about the nature of concepts in general rather than about particular concepts. (Although it has been possible to apply it to the concept of 'health' that is of central concern to us.) But context is important even in this apparently abstract argument. Within the first few paragraphs of his argument, Gallie is at pains to locate it within the wider sweep of the history of philosophy and in contemporary (for him) understanding of the limits of philosophy, in particular:

> Widespread [contemporary] repudiation of the idea of philosophy as a kind of 'engine' of thought, that can be laid on to eliminate conceptual confusions wherever they may arise. (Gallie, 1956: 168)

Gallie wants to present an argument laying claim to the capacity of philosophy to help resolve conceptual confusion; therefore he needs to point to the wider context of resistance to this idea, at least partly to demonstrate the boldness of his claim and his argument. So it's possible to see even highly abstract argument such as this taking place in a context.

Moreover, context provides important clues as to why a given argument is being developed, which in turn suggest reasons for critiquing it – and ultimately for deciding whether it is one we can or cannot support. In the case of the 'Saving Lives' example above, we might choose to base our critique on the separate conceptions of responsibility for health contained in this policy document and in earlier Conservative ones. Knowledge of context provides us with clear grounds for contrast. In the example of Gallie's 'essentially contested concepts', we might want to consider the realism of his argument in the context of general disdain of the belief that philosophy is some kind of never-failing 'cure-all' for problems of conceptual understanding. In both examples (and many others), context helps us to get going in our process of examination and critique.

Thinking Point

Consider a health studies-related argument you have been asked to analyse. How much do you know about its context? How might understanding its context contribute to your analysis and your eventual position in relation to the argument?

The Structure of Argument

All arguments – even weak arguments – possess a structure, which in turn frames content. The difference is that the structure of strong argument is clear and the content embodied within it is convincing. Of course, even if an argument is strong, this doesn't necessarily mean that we will be able to agree with its conclusions. For reasons that could be either rational or non-rational, we might reject it. We might, for example, be aware of evidence not considered in the argument we are analysing, and which seems to us to be compelling. Or we might stick to an alternative position through personal convictions, our own values, beliefs and ideologies. I'll discuss the relationship between values and argument in more detail later on. What's important is that we have engaged in critique of the argument, considered its strength and then formulated our own position based on careful critical analysis.

The most conventional structure of written argument is:

▸ *Introduction*, framing the *central idea* within the argument;
▸ *Detailed exposition* of the central idea, using *evidence* (empirical or theoretical or both) to support this;
▸ Consideration of possible *counter-arguments* and *counter-evidence*;
▸ *Conclusion* (Bonnett, 2001).

The importance of this kind of structure, and what makes it the structure of genuine *argument*, is its inclusion of alternative or contradictory positions – different positions to the one being advocated. The writer actively acknowledges and considers differences. These may not ultimately have any effect on the position they adopted at the beginning of their argument. However, seeking out evidence of a writer's willingness to understand and account for perspectives other than their own preferred one is a way in which we can begin critical analysis of argument.

We can do this in the first place by trying to get a sense of the argument's overall structure. If it follows something like the model above, we might start to get a feeling for the writer's concern (or not) to engage with different positions. It will perhaps begin to tell us something of their own stance and the degree of critical analysis contained within this.

Of course, this doesn't mean that we should dismiss work failing to conform to this broad structure of argument. If it doesn't seem to be apparent, we probably need to think about whether the work we are examining is trying to convince us of a position or an idea in a different kind of way – by claims to authority, perhaps. Then the question is whether the device of argument being used is acceptable to us, as well as whether it is appropriate (I will discuss the issue of argument by different means further on in this chapter.).

Thinking Point

Locate three health studies-related arguments, contained in material you have read. If you wish, you can use the arguments I've developed in the first four chapters of this book related to the three central components of 'the difficulty of health studies' (summarised on pages 92–94).

To what extent do they follow the structure of exposition and counter-argument I've described above? If they don't, what *is* their structure? What does this analysis of the arguments' *structures* begin to suggest to you about the nature and quality of the argument itself?

The Content of Argument: The 'Central Idea'

I talked just before about arguments containing some kind of 'central idea'. Such an idea is vital, because this is what drives the argument forward. It is, if you like, the nub of the 'story' that the writer is trying to tell, and to convince the reader about. The central idea of an argument may take a number of different forms. In essence, it will always be some kind of *thesis*, a statement that the writer intends to try and prove, or to advance (Marshall and Rowland, 1998). Within any argument, the thesis may take a number of different forms:

▸ *A bold (maybe even provocative) assertion.* What is being said is already a truth, it simply needs to be proved;
▸ *A specific question.* Asking this suggests that it would be interesting and important to find out more about the issue raised by the question;
▸ *A more general statement.* This might suggest that the broad area indicated by the statement, together with the difficulties, contradictions and tensions it contains, is worthwhile exploring (Bonnett, 2001).

Trying to work out what a writer's thesis (their central idea) actually is forms an important task for someone analysing an argument for two reasons:

▸ *We need to be sure that the argument is worth considering.* Health studies students have limited time available to them and so there is generally a need to focus on arguments that are important, rather than marginal. For example, an argument based on a central idea that health is disease absence *might* be more essential to review than one advancing the case that the health of individuals depends on faithful observation of the Summer Solstice. But here there is an important contingency; *does the argument have current relevance for us?* If we were particularly interested in the relationship between health beliefs and ancient cultures such as Druidism, say, then in fact the Summer Solstice argument might actually be an essential one to review.

▸ *We need to have a benchmark against which to scrutinise the argument as a whole.* The key question that the critical analyst of health-related argument needs to be asking all the time is: Does the evidence the writer is supplying contribute to effective consideration of the central idea he or she has said they intended to explore?

Thinking Point

Here are three extracts from the beginnings of randomly selected papers engaging in health studies-related argument:

Screening programmes are often started prematurely – an example is cervical cancer – and once such programmes have started they are very difficult to stop. Some health authorities and many general practitioners have already started population screening. Before uncontrolled screening expands further, a critical review of the evidence is needed. (Smith *et al.*, 1989: 372)

Health promotion is frequently said to proceed from the premise that *individuals are responsible for their health.* ... Fine – but what does it mean? Perhaps nothing more profound than that people will usually be healthier if they try to take better care of themselves. ... [Or it may be] understood as having moral and policy implications. ... In either case, it is important to explore the

Thinking Point   *continued*

meanings and implications of the concept of personal responsibility for health before enshrining it as the motto of a new school of health promotion and education. (Wikler, 1987: 11)

Our concern is that many of the "popular" models and theories of health-related behaviour such as the health belief model, the theory of reasoned action and the stages of change model – all of which purport to outline, describe or explain individual health action – can be interpreted in such a fashion as to reflect merely the ideological standpoint of the user. The result is a perpetuation of interpretational ambiguities regarding their role and function. (Brown and Piper, 1995: 115)

What is the *central idea*, the *thesis*, being expressed by each writer (or writing team) – the thesis you think will be explored in some way in the argument that follows? Write down your understanding of the thesis, *in your own words*. What kinds of *lines of enquiry* do you think the writers will need to pursue in order to engage with the thesis and prove to you their argument in relation to it?

This particular 'Thinking Point' has three purposes. First, it encourages you to consider the central idea within each of the arguments chosen. This may not prove as easy as might be thought, particularly if you're looking at the argument 'raw', rather than through an extract. I'd encourage you to do this (references all appear in the bibliography), because one of the difficulties in identifying an argument's central thesis is that it is often hidden in other issues and themes raised at the beginning of an argument. (I've made life easier for you here by using quotations from the writers' work that I think represent the essence of the thesis that each wants to explore!)

Second, the potential 'hiddenness' of the central idea or thesis is what lies behind me asking you to express your understanding of the thesis *in your own words*. Part of the problem of the mysteriousness and 'unteachability' of academic analysis lies in the fact that the language academics use often appears to be complex and obfuscating. What does, for instance 'A perpetuation of interpretational ambiguities regarding [health behaviour models' and theories'] role and function' actually *mean?* One tactic for dealing with this kind of situation is described by Creme and Lea (1997: 44). Instead of battling away with language and phraseology that may not make complete (or possibly any) sense to you, try to convert it into words that you do in fact use every day, words with which you are familiar and comfortable. So Brown and Piper's expression above might be converted into, 'People like academics and practitioners continue to think about theories and models of health behaviour in lots of different and confusing ways.' This sort of 'translation' work might well help you become clearer, in your own terms, about what the central idea or thesis of a particular argument actually is.

The third purpose of the 'Thinking Point' is to return us to what becomes the key reason for identifying an argument's central thesis. This is its use as a benchmark for scrutiny of the argument. We always need to ask ourselves the question, 'If this is the writer's central thesis, does the evidence being used support and justify it adequately? Is it appropriate? What are its shortcomings? Can we accept them or should we be concerned about them? And if we are concerned, does this mean that we have to reject the argument as a whole?

The Content of Argument: From Assertion to Evidence

I talked before of writers *asserting* their central ideas (theses) at the beginnings of their arguments. Each of the three statements in the 'Thinking Point' above can be understood as an assertion (or perhaps more than one assertion). That is, each is making a claim that such and such a thing is true, without at that moment having offered reasons (Fairbairn and Winch, 1998: 190). For example, we might suggest that Smith *et al.* (1989) are asserting the danger of uncontrolled health screening and therefore the need to examine evidence of the effectiveness and efficacy of screening before policy makers and practitioners continue with projects of mass screening.

Now we might in fact have some sympathy with this assertion. We might even believe that it is true as it stands; it does seem sensible to be worried about uncontrolled screening, and therefore support careful examination of screening policy and practices. But at the moment this is a position based on belief, not one emerging from a process of critical analysis. Smith and colleagues have so far presented no argument for their assertion, and no evidence supporting their argument.

The key tasks for those attempting to develop effective argument are:

▸ To build up their case using appropriate and convincing evidence;
▸ To identify weaknesses in the argument and evidence of others who hold contrary positions.

So the key tasks for the person critically analysing argument are:

▸ Assessment of the worth and value of evidence used in support of the central idea or thesis;

▸ Assessment of the extent to which the writer is justified in rejecting alternative positions (and the arguments and evidence that go with these).

Thinking Point

Fairbairn and Winch (1998: 188) talk of 'assertions posing as arguments'. By this they mean that a writer might put forward a series of assertions, offer no evidence to support them, yet still give the impression that they are *arguing* rather than *asserting*. They might do this, for example, by never making it clear that they are simply giving an opinion or expressing a belief.

While we might in fact agree with the assertions being made by the writer, we need to be wary of 'assertions posing as arguments'. *Why* is the writer unwilling or unable to point to evidence supporting their assertions? *Why* aren't they acknowledging that they are simply expressing an opinion or a belief?

Try and identify from your own health studies-related reading a piece that is 'assertion posing as argument'. Read it through again and ask yourself these questions in relation to the piece.

Those constructing health-related arguments use a range of different kinds of evidence in support of those arguments. This is hardly surprising, given the variety of potential focuses on 'health' that we might want to develop along with the presence of a range of different disciplinary interests – not to mention the contested nature of the concept itself. In Chapter 3, I began to distinguish between the different kinds of discourse used by the health-related disciplines to advance their arguments. I identified three broad kinds of discourse and argument: *empirical, analytic* and *normative*. Each kind of argument is based on evidence of one sort or another (or a combination of kinds of evidence).

Empirical argument is based on *empirical evidence*. That is, its argument that something, X, is the way that it is, is derived from evidence gained in some way through observation of 'the real world'. This kind of argument is frequently favoured in the field of health studies partly because, as I've discussed, the 'shadow of biomedicine' is cast over the whole field. Biomedicine and its disciplines have a strong affinity with quantitative methodologies and methods, designed to uncover objective empirical facts. The best known of these – the 'gold standard' of biomedical research – is the Randomised Controlled Trial (RCT). The RCT conforms to the principles of experimental design (Tones and Green, 2004). The effects of an intervention are observed through those subject to the intervention (the experimental group) being closely monitored. A further group not receiving the intervention (the control group) is also closely observed. The difference in effect between the experimental group and the control group is thus attributed to the intervention.

A variety of other quantitative methodologies and methods aspire to this 'gold standard' of objectivism. But those aspiring to interpretivist positions on health also very often rely on empirical observation of one sort or another to frame their arguments. (See, for example, Cornwell, 1984; Blackburn, 1991; Wilson-Barnett and Macleod-Clark, 1993; Bunton, Nettleton and Burrows, 1995.) It's possible to claim, then, that much argument in the field of health studies is based on empirical evidence, although the extent to which it's used and how it operates alongside other kinds of evidence will vary between arguments, as I'll discuss.

Analytic argument attempts to explain not only *how* but also *why* something is the way that it is. Clearly it's possible for analytic argument to draw on empirical evidence as part of this kind of project. However, it might also use other sorts of evidence. An analytic argument for viewing health as a human good, for example, would examine the component parts of the idea of 'health'. This might involve accounts of health drawn from individuals (empirical evidence); but it might also draw on more theoretical kinds of evidence. It could, for example, use theological or philosophical constructions of personhood as part of an attempt to demonstrate the necessary connection between being a whole person and being healthy (so moving to the conclusion that 'health' is a human good or value). The combination of the use of empirical and theoretical evidence is what helps advance the argument further into the territory of 'Why?' and not just 'How?'

Normative argument might equally draw on both empirical and theoretical evidence. Normative argument is argument *based on prescribed norms and standards*, which have already been assumed prior to the formulation of the argument concerned. So again, for example, a norm or standard that might be assumed in an argument for viewing health as a human good might be that it contributes to human welfare. Importantly, this norm is not debated within the argument. It is already there, embedded, and used as one of the foundations for the argument that health should be seen as a human good. But the norm, it's presumed, will have been based on evidence of some kind: perhaps empirical (observation that in general, societies with greater levels of health flourish better); or perhaps theoretical (the kinds of evidence that might be cited in an analytic argument for health as a human good). The normative argument may also, of course, use both empirical and theoretical evidence to support its claims, and possibly also to support the norms and standards that it has already assumed. In both cases, the evidence requires analysis and, if necessary, challenge. It's especially important to look for evidence supporting the assumed norms, if it exists within the argument. There's a need to be aware that very often in normative argument, evidence for assumptions with regard to norms and standards may be thin or even non-existent within the argument itself. The writer, after all, is assuming these. But this shouldn't stop us from disagreeing with the assumptions if we think we ought to do so.

Writers, in developing their arguments, may not necessarily stick to just one kind. Indeed, it's probable that they won't. Arguments are very often complex and multilayered, using a variety of devices to move them along. Getting to grips potentially with a mix of types of argumentation poses yet another challenge for the critical analyst. The author of the argument might well present, say, an argument based substantially on empirical evidence, but which contains strong normative assumptions. For example, a lengthy review of the most effective health promotion options for reducing smoking (Reid *et al.*, 1992) involves examination of evidence in relation to the subject, resulting in more than 120 citations. The paper concludes with the following remark:

> The former Chief Medical Officer for England, Sir George Godber, said of the smoking epidemic in 1983: "Future generations would be aghast that we did so little." If we are to avoid the censure both of Sir George and our grandchildren, the single most important task is to win the battle for public opinion. Without popular support, there will be neither effective fiscal policy nor mandatory advertising controls; neither will there be adequate funding for health promotion. (Reid *et al.*, 1992: 193–194)

Reid and his colleagues are presenting an argument strongly based on empirical evidence for the effectiveness of certain measures to prevent smoking. But they are also making at least one normative assumption (interestingly held back until the very end of their argument); namely, that smoking prevention is a worthwhile activity. Of course, we might well agree with this assumption. There are certainly very strong imperatives to do so. However, we are also free to disagree. (See, for example, the argument *against* smoking prevention advanced by Skrabanek and McCormick (1989) which also, inevitably, contains normative assumptions.) In the case of something like the argument from Reid and colleagues, the requirement on us as critical analysts is not to take any argument at face value. Here, we should not accept that because this argument contains lots of 'real world' evidence, it must be wholly an argument from empiricism. We need to try and establish whether assumptions are being made – or more likely *what* assumptions exist – and then determine if we agree or disagree with them.

Thinking Point

Consider again the beginning of each of the three arguments contained in the Thinking Point on page 105–106 (Smith *et al.*, Wikler and Brown and Piper). From these beginnings, what *kind* of argument would you expect them to develop (based on my heuristic division between empirical, analytic and normative)? What *sort* of evidence would you expect them to produce in support of their arguments? (If you have specific ideas of possible evidence – for example, that you would expect Smith *et al.* to produce evidence of the effectiveness or otherwise of particular kinds of screening programmes – note these down.)

The idea I'm trying to develop now is that it's possible to establish a set of general heuristics – rules of thumb – for examining health-related argument. Importantly, this has not been borrowed or imported from a particular discipline, but actually emerges from our own careful study of the field and the nature of the arguments it contains.

Identifying this possibility is key. Earlier I discussed the difficulties engendered for us by separate disciplines operating according to their own sets of heuristics. Because we are students of an *interdisciplinary* field of health studies, we may not be familiar in detail (or even at all) with the heuristics of a particular discipline – sociology, say. As a result, we may be anxious about our capacity to examine (let alone to challenge) a health-related argument emerging from that particular discipline. But it's precisely because we're involved in a *field* of study that we can develop our own set of procedures for analysing argument. We can begin to identify common themes and features of health-related arguments from across the range of disciplines and start to establish principles for their examination; ways of working out which arguments are good or bad, and which are acceptable or unacceptable to us.

It's important to be clear at this point about both the possibilities and the limits of the evolving idea that we can construct a set of heuristics for the study of health. On the one hand, recognition and consideration of 'the difficulty of health studies', its roots and nature, reasonably leads us to a belief in the importance of critical analysis (and of critical reflection) in understanding and dealing with the problems brought about by a highly disputable concept. So developing a set of heuristics, through analysis and reflection, for dealing with disagreement and debate seems to be a worthwhile project.

On the other hand, the project shouldn't go too far. I don't want to suggest that we can, or should, rely completely on what some might see as generic and generalised skills in dealing with the difficulties of conceptual and practical understanding raised by the idea of 'health'. Certainly we can use the generic tools of analysis and reflection to help us here. But we need to do so carefully. And we must complement this use with attempts to understand the contributions (both helpful and confusing) of particular disciplines with regard to health. To this extent, we need to immerse ourselves in a sustained encounter with the disciplines – with the different assumptions they make as well as the beliefs they hold and the sets of heuristics by which they operate.

Argument, Values and Authority

Before I clarify and summarise what might be involved in a set of heuristics for critical analysis in the field of health studies, there are a number of further aspects of the nature of argument to be considered. Much of the focus of this chapter has been on the analysis of argument that possesses a specific kind of structure (argument, counter-argument and its assessment, conclusion). However, there's a need to consider other kinds of arguments.

Broadly, the sort of argument we've been examining so far is what we might call *rational* argument. It is rational at least partly because it attempts to provide substantiation in the form of evidence of one sort or another for the assertions that it is making. It moves from assertion to evidence to considering possible counter-evidence and then to its conclusion. But it is rational also because it does not attempt to persuade by appealing, one way or another, to our non-rational side (Fairbairn and Winch, 1998). This sounds like a truism; an argument is rational if it appeals to our rationality! So I need to be clear about what I mean by 'non-rationality' in the first place, and then relate it to my arguments for 'the difficulty of health studies'.

It seems fairly easy to recognise that we are all subject to arguments that rely for at least some of their effect on appeal to our emotions. This seems especially so in the political world. This chapter was being written in the summer of 2005. Whenever I took a break from work and turned on the news or read the papers, two stories dominated the political headlines. One was the proposed introduction of identity (ID) cards in the United Kingdom. The other was the attempt to get much greater commitment on the part of the rich industrialised nations (the so-called G8) to dealing compassionately with Third World debt and poverty – the 'Make Poverty History' campaign. The more I heard about these two stories, the more it seemed to me that both the ID card and the anti-poverty campaigners were using, at least in part, non-rational means to carry forward their arguments, although in different ways and for different effects. The ID card campaigners (the government and its supporters) were certainly drawing on empirical evidence and using some rational means to persuade people of their case. For example, they pointed to the effect that ID cards had in other countries in successfully combating things like social security fraud. However, there seemed no doubt that they were also using non-rational means to advance their case. In particular, there were many attempts (mostly never at all explicit) at emotional persuasion. Our fears, for example, were being played on by frequent references to the use of ID cards in protecting national security and thwarting terrorist attack. Of course, the campaigners against ID cards were similarly using non-rational argument based on emotional persuasion – exploitation of the issue of the erosion of personal liberty, for example, was founded partly on fear.

The anti-poverty campaigners were also making use of empirical evidence and rational means to support their argument – statistics about indebtedness, about global inequalities in the wealth of nations and so on were often being used in what I heard and read. But again these arguments were underscored by appeals to emotion. How could rich nations be so selfish? How could we tolerate so much suffering on the part of others? And so on.

Why were both of these arguments using non-rational means of persuasion, particularly it seems in the form of appeals to emotion? There are probably many reasons, some of which we might be able to agree with and others that we wouldn't. But I think there are two that are especially worth pointing to, each strongly connected to the other:

▸ In each example, the arguments are essentially about *values*. Values involved include personal liberty, national security, global responsibility, even the value of humanity and being human itself. This is hardly surprising, given that politics is essentially about values and that political policy is the authoritative allocation of values (Easton, 1953). As I've already argued, dispute and disagreement about values is particularly acrimonious. This is partly because such dispute can't be settled by simple recourse to the facts. Here, those arguing for ID cards or for combating global poverty attempted to promote their values partly by suggesting that we should all hold those values. They were unable to do this just by pointing to 'the evidence', whatever that is, simply because it couldn't play an irrefutable part in our acceptance or rejection of values. So they had to make recourse to other means of persuasion, which in these examples seems to me to have included emotional persuasion.

▸ In both examples, the issues that are being dealt with are simply *too large* for their advocates (and adversaries) to convey in narrow empirical or analytic terms. A wholly analytic argument for, say, the eradication of global poverty would be hugely extensive. It would also be missing much of the point of the debate. One of the important things those arguing in favour of ID cards and global poverty reduction alike want to get across is that we should simply *just accept* their arguments. They are so essential, so intrinsically *right* that we would be denying our common sense if we were to reject them. They embody the *values* of the campaigners and so demand our interest, respect and acceptance. (And of course that is the point where this second reason and the first meet, in a movement beyond facts and analysis to judgement based on values.)

This idea of the 'rightness' of a particular argument leads us to the idea of the *argument from authority* (Bonnett, 2001: 104). In this kind of argument, we are being asked to accept something is so mainly because a particular authority says that it is the case. In the examples that we've just been considering, the government (those elected in sufficient numbers to control the affairs of our state) asserts it has enough authority to determine that the introduction of ID cards will enhance our security and statehood without detrimental effect to our liberty. And the 'Make Poverty History' campaigners are equally asserting that they represent sufficiently the concerns of ordinary people, combined with their own expertise and that of supportive academics and policy analysts, to argue authoritatively for changed approaches from the 'G8' politicians.

The use of these examples draws the distinction nicely made by Fairbairn and Winch (1998: 205) between the arguments of those who are *in authority* and those who are *an authority*. Fairbairn and Winch reasonably claim that simply because someone or some group is in a position of authority does not make them an expert on the subject in question. In terms of my examples, it might be possible to argue that the 'G8' politicians (*in authority*) do not necessarily possess the expertise of the 'Make Poverty History' coalition, an individual member of which might be regarded as *an authority* on the subject concerned. Regardless, though, of the source from which an argument from authority emerges, the simple fact that it comes from authority – someone or some organisation asserting that their claims should be accepted – does not mean by itself that we should accept those claims. If a critically analytic perspective is to be maintained, we need to engage in the same rigorous consideration as we would with other kinds of argument. There may be good reasons for accepting arguments based on non-rational grounds (including those appealing to emotions, or attempting to influence from authority). But we need to be completely clear what those reasons are.

Thinking Point

What, for you, would be *good* reasons for accepting an argument based on non-rational grounds? What would be *poor* reasons?

If all this seems to be drawing us away from health-related discussions, I want to suggest that the opposite is the case. I've already argued strongly for the crucial contribution of values towards 'the difficulty of health studies'. If values are an important reason for engaging in non-rational argument, then we can probably expect that such argument features frequently in our field. Equally, if we agree with the idea that authority (especially medical authority) plays a large part in determining how views and directions on 'health' are formed and pursued, it follows that we need to keep a close watch on arguments from authority within our field. Do we agree with them? Can they be justified?

Thinking Point

The following are summaries of two health-related arguments that I would characterise as arguments from authority. I'd encourage you to read the complete argument if you can, but if this isn't possible, rely on these summaries to address the questions that follow them.

Argument 1

Scally and Donaldson (1998: 61–65) reflect on the 'New' Labour government's requirement that clinical governance is to be the main vehicle driving quality in the NHS following its first election victory. They argue that clinical governance demands changes in organisational structure: that local professional self-regulation will be the key to dealing with problems of poor performance amongst NHS clinicians; and that new approaches are required with regard to the recognition and dissemination of good clinical practice. At the time of their writing, both authors were in influential management positions in the NHS. (Donaldson later became the Chief Medical Officer for England and Wales.)

Argument 2

Ackroyd (1984: 147) rejects the claim by two academics, Sider and Clements (1984), that patients have a moral obligation to preserve their own health and thus to follow their doctors' medical advice. She argues instead that a more equal partnership between doctor and patient, rather than the paternalistic model advocated by Sider and Clements, is likely to result in a genuinely common interest being pursued. At the time of writing, Ackroyd was the Chair of the Patient's Association, a national voluntary body aiming to promote the interests of patients.

In relation to each of these arguments:

▸ Would you regard the argument as being proposed by individuals who are *in* authority, or who are *an* authority?
▸ What would be your reasons for accepting (or rejecting) each of these arguments from authority?

Procedures for Critically Analysing Health-Related Arguments: A 'Rough Guide'

Finally I'm in a position to clarify and summarise my own set of procedures for critically analysing health studies-related arguments. These are my ideas of a set of heuristics, 'rules of thumb', to point us in the right direction for dealing with the complex arguments and debate that exist in the field of interest to us. They are, I suppose, the beginnings of my own 'rough guide' to making sense of the field's complex territory. But like the real 'Rough Guides', those incredibly helpful guides to travelling in unfamiliar cities and countries, the beginning of my own 'rough guide' should be prefaced with a warning. What I'm clarifying here is a set of generalised principles and procedures for dealing with some aspects of 'the difficulty of health studies'. I hope they have uses, but they also have limits. In particular, they need to be accompanied by a commitment to immersing ourselves in a sustained encounter with the disciplines themselves that contribute to shaping and understanding conceptions of health. The 'Rough Guide' to Paris is fine – in fact it's very useful – but you won't know what Paris is really like until you've actually been there!

Stages in Critically Analysing Health-Related Argument

Stage 1: Understanding and Analysing the Argument's Context

What is the context of the argument? Has the argument you are analysing explicitly described and/or discussed the relationship between context and the argument now being presented? If so, what effect has this had in terms of building up the argument? If the context hasn't been explicitly described and/or discussed, why do you think this is so?

Stage 2: Identifying, Understanding and Analysing the Argument's Structure

What is the structure of the argument you are considering? Does it follow the 'conventional' structure of academic argument, discussed earlier? If it doesn't, why is this so? Is the lack of conventional argument/counter-argument structure acceptable? (See Stage 5, below.)

Stages in Critically Analysing Health-Related Argument *continued*

Stage 3: Identifying, Understanding and Analysing the Argument's 'Central Idea'

What is the argument's 'central idea', or thesis? Is it of relevance/interest to you at this point in your study of health? Why? If it isn't, are there still reasons for considering it?

Stage 4: Understanding and Analysing the Argument's Content

Does the argument you are considering contain evidence for the claims being made? Does it consider possible counter evidence? (If not, it has failed to move from assertion to argument and although we might agree with the assertion, neither the writer nor ourselves have justified our beliefs.)

Is the argument empirical, analytic or normative (or a combination)? Is the evidence offered in support of the argument (theoretical/empirical) convincing? Does the argument contain *assumptions?* Are these explicit or implicit? If explicit, are they justified and is that justification adequate? If they are implicit, why do you think this is so? Can we agree with such implicit assumptions?

Stage 5: Understanding and Analysing Non-Rational Influences within Arguments

Does the argument appear to have a non-rational element? How strong is this? What is the nature of this element (e.g., does it contain appeal to emotions, or attempt to argue from authority)? What values underpin any non-rational argument or element of argument that you are considering? Can you agree with those values? Can you (do you *have* to) agree with the authority contained in any argument from authority that you encounter?

Turning Point?

This Turning Point simply asks you to adopt a critically analytic perspective on the the project on which I've embarked, which will continue in the next chapter – the creation of a set of heuristics to be used in arguments encountered within the field of health

Turning Point? *continued*

studies. To what extent do you think it is likely to support your own sense – making with regard to the complex and contested arguments that abound in the field? Is it just too simplistic to imagine that a set of 'rules' such as I've begun to develop can help with sorting out the competing values and ideologies, the different styles of argumentation, the separate sorts of evidence that are used in health studies-related arguments? Whether or not you agree with the kind of project I'm involved in, it is important that your judgement comes as a result of deliberative analysis rather than an unsubstantiated 'point of view'.

What's gone on in this chapter?

In this chapter, I have developed an account of the nature of critical analysis as a process for examining the arguments we are likely to encounter in the field of health studies. I've described and discussed the essential importance of argument and its analysis in the 'applied' field of health studies. Our acceptance or rejection of arguments will potentially make a real difference to others. There is thus a need to be as clear as possible about the worth of particular arguments and to develop skills in recognising and critiquing both *how* and *why* they have been constructed. Although it holds important limitations, there is use in developing, as I've done at the end of this chapter, a 'set of procedures' for the investigation and analysis of health-related argument.

6 Health Studies and Critical Reflection

What is this chapter going to do?

Having discussed the process of critical *analysis*, I now move on to considering the process of critical *reflection*. It is as essential for the health studies student to engage in reflection as it is in analysis. I argue that the processes are fundamentally connected and we can't be said to be committing ourselves to 'whole person' learning if we neglect one or the other. We need analysis to critique the supposedly rational arguments within the field of health studies; and we need reflection to help understand the beliefs and values that underlie argument and our reaction to it. I describe and discuss a model of reflection, and how we can engage in reflective processes, paying particular attention to the importance of writing in supporting and developing reflective capacity. Finally, I add to the 'rough guide' I began at the end of the last chapter, suggesting a set of principles for engaging in health studies-related reflection.

Developing the Connection between Critical Analysis and Critical Reflection

The capacity to engage in effective analysis of argument is an essential one for the health studies student to develop. Equally important is the ability to engage in the process of critical reflection. I want to begin this chapter by clarifying the nature of the connection between critical analysis and critical reflection. Doing so will serve to emphasise that one or other of these processes on its own is not enough to tackle the problems that are apparent in the field of health studies. We need both.

Thinking Point

Before reading further, review the discussion in the previous chapter on the nature of critical analysis and its place in examining health studies related arguments. From this, what do you think are the *limits* of critical *analysis* in the study of health? From your awareness of the process of critical *reflection*, how could it help extend our understanding beyond these limits?

Critical analysis ('technical rationality'), I argue, can't form the whole of our response to 'the difficulty of health studies'. This is because of:

▸ The nature of health-related argument itself;

▸ And because of what is involved in our reactions to, and learning from, such argument.

Limits to Critical Analysis and the Importance of Critical Reflection: The Nature of Health-Related Argument

'Health' is a contested and disputed concept. Given this, it follows that wholly rational, analytic argument about its nature, while essential, can only go so far. Continuing with an example from the previous chapter we can analyse Smith *et al.*'s (1989) argument against population screening of blood cholesterol levels (a risk factor for coronary heart disease (CHD)) in the United Kingdom. We can examine the empirical claims that he and his colleagues make about the logistics of screening in the British context and of follow-up of those at risk. At least in principle, these claims can be verified or disputed. We can connect these claims to others within the argument and assess its worth and force overall. But even though we might think that many of the claims made in the argument are factually correct, and that it is carefully and forcefully constructed, *we can still disagree with its outcome.*

If we do so, our position won't simply be bloody-minded. It will be based instead, perhaps, on our own particular conceptions of the nature of health. We might believe that 'health' at least partly involves fewer people becoming prey to CHD. Therefore we need to support screening programmes that aim to reduce heart disease. We will be disagreeing with Smith and his colleagues. Alternatively, we might believe that 'health' involves not encouraging people to subject themselves to procedures that could be indeterminate in their outcome and so cause worry and concern (Marteau, 1990; Skrabanek, 1990). So we support Smith *et al.*'s concern about screening. Both of these positions, resulting in either agreement or disagreement with Smith and colleagues, could be regarded as reasonable. They have both stemmed from the same argument and the same set of facts. That both are possible relates in part to the disputability of ideas about the nature of health.

As this example shows, dispute and contest over the nature of the concept of health means that no matter how apparently watertight a health-related argument is, there will always be the opportunity to disagree with it, and to do so not simply for reasons of perversity. Critical analysis will take us a good distance in understanding and dealing with health-related argument, but not the whole way.

Thinking Point

'No matter how apparently watertight a health-related argument is, it will always be possible to disagree with it ... .'

On the basis of the discussions and arguments presented so far in this book, together with your own reactions and perceptions, can you agree with my assertion?

Limits to Critical Analysis and the Importance of Critical Reflection: Dealing with Beliefs and Values

This leads on to the idea that the use of critical analysis in considering the arguments of health studies is limited to some degree because of what is involved in our reactions to, and our learning from, such arguments. In the CHD screening example I've been discussing, I have claimed that we might regard both eventual positions on the argument as reasonable. Ultimately, though, we will take up one or the other position because it aligns more closely with our own set of *beliefs*. In this example, we might consider our beliefs not only about the nature of health but also, say, about the efficacy of prevention and the worth of an essentially medical approach to this area as we decide which position to adopt.

The range of beliefs that might be invoked in our reaction to the CHD screening argument is potentially much wider. Each belief is likely to be accompanied by a corresponding value. For example, if I believed in the worth of this kind of screening and the important role of medically oriented health services in preventing disease (and so promoting health) in this way, I would hold particular views on the nature of the value of health. I would also regard the value of health care and its role in determining and influencing peoples' lives in certain sorts of ways. In sum, the set of beliefs (and associated values) with which I encounter this kind of argument is likely to be influential and powerful.

Given the power and influence of beliefs and values within the argument, it's likely that they will play a large part in how we respond to it. Critical analysis, as I have argued, involves the development, under-standing and critique of reasoning and argument. There is clearly a gap between the scope of such analysis and the nature of argument in health studies as I've just described and discussed it. In this gap are the beliefs and values that form an essential part of the landscape of health studies. And it is this particular part of the landscape – beliefs and values – that is the focus of critical reflection (Boud, Keogh and Walker, 1985; Tate, 2004).

The connection between critical analysis and critical reflection in the context of health studies now becomes clearer:

▸ *Analysis* should enable us to dissect the supposedly rational arguments about health and what needs to be done to improve it that emerge from the disciplines feeding the field.
▸ *Reflection* allows us to move beyond this wholly rational examina-tion to consider how our beliefs and values influence our decisions about which arguments we should accept, or reject.

Reflection allows us to contemplate our reactions to the normative positions assumed within very many health-related arguments. It also allows us to consider our relationship with arguments that seek to influence by means such as appeals to authority. These kinds of con-templation and consideration are essential, given the nature of health and health care. So in our study of health, we need to engage in work that is both analytic and reflective. We need to involve ourselves, from Claxton (1988), in 'whole person learning'.

Reflecting on Theory, on Practice and on Learning

What is the scope of critical reflection in the field of health and health studies? There is perhaps a tendency to associate critical reflection predominantly with practice, to suggest that as a 'skill', its uses lie mainly in helping us to understand our professional actions and reactions. As a result of reflection, it's possible for us to improve what we do in the context of professional practice. This association of reflection mainly with practice is reinforced by the ways in which language is used in the area. As O'Connor *et al.* (2003) note, 'reflection' and 'reflective practice' are terms that are used interchangeably. This primary association might also emerge as a result of health care professions' concerns to ensure that those under their jurisdiction develop as 'reflective practitioners' (Powell, 1999), a phenomenon I discussed in Chapter 4. In the light of this, it's important to emphasise that the scope of critical reflection in the field of health and health studies embraces not only practice and practice-related learning but also conceptual and theoretical learning, as well as the learning process itself. In other words, health studies students need to engage in critical reflection on theory, on practice and on learning. They need to do so not least because they are all connected with and dependent on each other.

There are two reasons for suggesting this. First, if we accept an account of critical reflection which asserts that it is about evaluating and possibly offering solutions to problems of practice (Young, 2004), surely we have to consider as part of this theory that might be related to the practical problem. Schön argues that contexts encouraging reflection need to support the connection between what he calls 'general knowledge' (theory) and particular problematic cases (Schön, 1987: 39). Such contexts, he continues to argue should also support the development in understanding of *how* we learn about the theory-practice relationship and how we exploit both theory and practice to understand novel situations and improve our effectiveness in dealing with them. So learning from both practice and theory, and learning about such learning, are all interwoven in processes of critical reflection.

The second reason for suggesting the interdependent, interwoven nature of practice and learning in health studies-related critical reflection links to the ideas I've been developing about the kind of field we are involved with. In the previous chapter, I argued strongly for the practical relevance of theoretical analysis in our field because it is an 'applied' one. Our theoretical discussions and debates will have implications for what we do and how we behave in our everyday occupational and professional lives. I argue now that the inverse of this is also true. Our occupational and professional lives will help to shape and refine our understanding of theoretical discussion and debate. Let me return briefly to my earlier example (from Chapter 2) of the Nursing Process and report-writing. What I was trying to do here was to exemplify theoretical accounts of the so-called hidden curriculum. In turn the use of both this practical example and the theoretical idea contributed to my overall argument that our professional beliefs and values profoundly influence our understanding of 'health'. So it's possible to see how aspects of our occupational and professional lives can help to illuminate theoretical discussion Again this emphasises the connected nature of practice and theory in critical reflection related to the study of health. These connections are strongly represented, too, in health studies-related curriculum requirements of the Quality Assurance Agency for Higher Education (QAA) (Quality Assurance Agency for Higher Education, 2001).

Thinking Point

My purpose in emphasising the fundamental connections between theory and practice, and between these things and the process of learning, is so that they are all taken account of as a picture of critical reflection in the context of health studies is built up. Try and identify an incident from your own experience in which:

▸ You learnt something from health studies-related theory, which then seemed to be exemplified in your health-related practice AND/OR;
▸ You learnt something from your practice, which seemed to be represented in theory you'd encountered.

In either or both sort of incident, try also to recollect *how* you engaged in the learning that you experienced.

Health and The Process of Critical Reflection

I've now mapped out the nature of the connection between critical analysis and critical reflection, arguing that engaging in both processes allows us to extend our understanding and awareness beyond the 'technical-rational' and to embrace 'professional artistry' as well (using Schön's terms). In the context of my argument for 'the difficulty of health studies', the development of capacities with regard to both analysis and reflection should allow us to increase our understanding of the complex theoretical and empirical accounts we are presented with. It should also help us to understand our reactions to these. We should be able to respond to the problems of health studies not only in technical terms, but also in terms of the beliefs and values we encounter in the field – and that we hold ourselves. As I've argued, it is this complex amalgam of the rational and the ideological that fuels the dispute and disagreement inherent within the study of health.

Engaging in critical reflection as well as critical analysis, then, is likely to move us forward in 'whole person' understanding of health. It should support our self-development in the cause of desirable and effective practice (Tate, 2004). The central question now is one of how we work towards becoming critically reflective.

Reflection as an Everyday Process

Much has been written about the nature of professional reflection. (See, for example, the wide range of references appearing in Tate and Sills' (2004) recent review of the area.) Its philosophical underpinnings are substantial (Dewey, 1974; Schön, 1983, 1987). Maybe this makes professional reflection appear rather intimidating. But we need to remember that reflection is an everyday thing and not only a rarefied professional activity. Clearly there are particular ways of conceptualising and practising reflection in professional contexts; but emphasising that quite similar processes go on in our 'ordinary' lives might help to demystify the subject a little.

In a brief deflection from our 'health' focus, I want to go back to the creative writing example from Chapter 3 to help make my point about the everyday nature of reflection. I talked in that example about trying to get better at creative writing by going to evening classes, practising what I'd been taught, reading the published work of notable creative writers and so on. I would probably use a wide variety of methods to try and improve my skills in this area, but I would also most likely go through the process of improvement in a certain kind of way. I wouldn't move carelessly from one thing to another. What I would do would be to formulate some kind of plan (at least in my head) before doing anything.

At various points I would probably review my progress and possibly amend the plan (again if only in my head). Imagine that I'd gone to one term of the evening class and found it really helpful to talk to others with the same interest as me and to a tutor who was experienced in the area. It would be more than likely that I'd sign up for another term or possibly (if I was really keen) look at joining a second class run by the same tutor. Or maybe I thought that the evening class was too much geared towards a certain type of writing (radio script writing, say), which wasn't my main interest. Perhaps other members of the class were difficult to get on with, or the tutor's advice was obscure. Then I might look around for another class. Alternatively, I might think about why this one was proving difficult and identify things that I could do or different ways that I might behave with the aim of making it better and improving my experience of it. The point is that at this stage in my project of getting better at creative writing, I would be actively evaluating my experience and changing or reinforcing my plans as appropriate. I would be doing so in a way that somehow allowed me to assess the experience, what I was learning, how I felt about it and how it connected to what else I was doing to try and improve my skill. I would be thinking about my thinking. In other words, in this example (as well as in lots of others from everyday life) I would be *reflecting*.

Thinking Point

Consider your everyday, non-professional or non-academic life. Identify an aspect of it where you've actively sought to improve your skills. This might be a hobby or a sport, or a family-oriented activity of some kind – it doesn't matter, so long as it's not professional or academic. Think about the process that you've gone through to improve those skills. Does it match at all with the kind of process described in my creative writing example? Would you agree with my describing this kind of process as one of *reflection?*

The Central Components of Reflection-on-Action

I want to draw again the distinction I made in Chapter 4 between reflection-*on-action* on the one hand; and reflection-*in-action* on the other:

▸ *Reflection-on-action* is the process whereby the individual engages reflectively with a learning-or practice-related incident at some point after it has actually taken place;

▸ *Reflection-in-action* involves engagement in reflective processes while we are actually in the particular incident concerned.

For Benner (1984) among others, this latter reflective process is the mark of the expert practitioner. (And it's possible to suggest that it's the mark of the expert *learner*, too.) It is intuitive, its key distinction from reflection-on-action being that it has immediate significance for the incident because we are able to change what we are doing while there is still the opportunity to make a difference there and then (Schön, 1987: 29).

It is true that our ultimate goal might be to become skilled in reflection-in-action to become expert practitioners and expert learners. But we still need to learn how it is possible to reflect *on* our action first. We need to know how we can encourage processes that allow us to use the situations of practice and learning we've encountered in the past in such a way that we understand them better – and eventually we are helped to deal with 'new' situations (Schön, 1987: 39). My focus, in the rest of this chapter, is directed towards understanding reflection-*on*-action.

I argue that the idea of using past situations to help us deal better with possible future ones implies three central components to the process of reflection-on-action:

▸ We need to have had the experience;
▸ We need to be able to look back at it in ways that enable us to make sense of it and understand it more deeply;
▸ We need to be able to use this retrospective understanding to fashion new and more effective ways of acting for the future.

These three components draw us back to the model of reflection (Figure 1) that I briefly presented in Chapter 4 and which I'll now discuss in more detail.

The Experience

Beginning with the experience, it's important for the reflective learner to allow themselves to be as open as possible to the situations they are encountering. There is a need, to some extent at least, to relish the prospect of spending time in what Schön calls 'the swampy lowland' of professional practice (within which we can include professional learning) where 'messy, confusing problems defy technical solution'

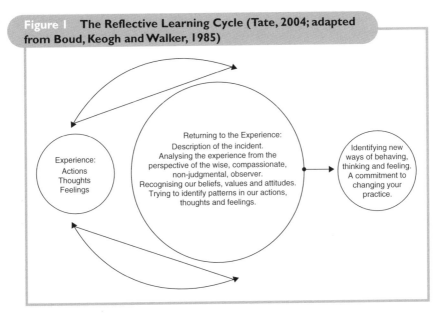

Figure 1   The Reflective Learning Cycle (Tate, 2004; adapted from Boud, Keogh and Walker, 1985)

Experience:
Actions
Thoughts
Feelings

Returning to the Experience:
Description of the incident.
Analysing the experience from the
perspective of the wise, compassionate,
non-judgmental, observer.
Recognising our beliefs, values and attitudes.
Trying to identify patterns in our actions,
thoughts and feelings.

Identifying new
ways of behaving,
thinking and feeling.
A commitment to
changing your
practice.

(Schön, 1987: 3). This openness to difficulty isn't perverse; it's a requirement of professionals learning and operating in an immensely complex world where simple rule-prescribing and following isn't enough to deal with difficulties.

The experience on which we decide to reflect might be an encounter with an aspect of theory, or it could be an incident from practice. Again, it could be a situation where theory and practice seem somehow to be linked together. (This is an important possibility given the argument I've just presented for the strong connection between the two in the field of health studies.) All of these kinds of experiences can contribute to learning about and understanding health.

The idea of being open to experience needs emphasis and explanation. There is a tendency, in professional action and learning, to view and understand experience in what we might describe as purely *cognitive* terms. What do we *know* and *think* about the action, whatever it is? This is perhaps especially so in the context of learning, where there is often a huge assumption that we need to operate strictly according to 'rational-technical' models of understanding. Take, for example, one of the initial ideas in this book – health as 'the absence of disease'. In coming across this idea, it's highly possible that in the first place we will try and 'order' it in our thoughts and in relation to our existing knowledge. We will attempt to focus on the idea alone and how it connects to other ideas and theories with which we are familiar. It's likely that we won't respond (or don't think we are responding) in anything other than this cognitive way.

Of course, this kind of cognitive response is important, as well as being what academics encourage. But if we are to engage in genuine reflection on the idea, to move beyond technical analysis alone, then we need to try and take account not simply of what we do and what we think. We also need to take account of how we *feel* about what we are encountering and our responses to those encounters. Thus feelings accompany actions and thoughts in the construction of the reflective learning cycle contained in the model in Figure 1.

But how is it possible to 'separate out' feelings from thoughts and actions within experience in the way that the model presented might imply? The short answer is that it's not. Remember that this is a model –a much simplified representation of reality. In truth, our feelings, thoughts and actions are interconnected in highly complex ways. Feelings, for example, have a profound influence on our motivation to act and on our cognitive processes (Tate, 2004). What is important at this stage of learning through reflection, the stage of experience, is a commitment to maintaining openness to that experience – what it evoked in terms of *feelings* as well as thoughts and actions – and to understanding it.

Return to the Experience

This leads to the second stage within the reflective cycle, the stage of returning to the experience. Openness to all aspects of experience would have little point unless we are also committed to understanding and analysing it as far as possible. So analysis needs to embrace thoughts, feelings and actions. We need to describe the experience and try to understand it as a 'whole person'. It's necessary to actively recognise our beliefs, values and attitudes, to connect these to what we've experienced, and in doing so try to form a complete picture of what we did and thought and felt. In turn, this will move us closer to answering the question of *why* we acted and thought and felt as we did.

This demanding task of 'whole person' analysis of their experience constitutes reflection-on-action. Because the reflection is *on* action, it is *a deliberative* process (in contrast to reflection-*in*-action, which is *intuitive*). As a process of deliberation, at least two things are needed:

▸ *Space* (mental and emotional as well as physical) in which to make sense of the complexity of our thoughts and feelings and actions;

▶ *Distance* from the experience. With distance comes a stronger possibility of seeing the experience with a degree of detachment, of taking on the role of the 'wise, compassionate, non-judgmental observer of our own experience' (Tate, 2004:13).

In talking of creating a distance between the experience and its analysis, I mean a distance of *time*. However, as the length of time can't be prescribed I also don't want to suggest that the gap between experience and point of analysis should be cleared of all thought about the experience itself and become a kind of blank no-mans-land. In particular there is a need as soon as possible after the incident to record details; what happened, what was being thought, what was being felt. I'll discuss how this might be done in the next section, along with how space might be created for reflection.

Let's consider an example to demonstrate the importance of creating space and distance in order to allow us the opportunity properly to reflect on academic understanding, practice experience, and the connection between the two. It's the idea of health as 'the absence of disease', as represented in the argument of JG Scadding, reviewed at various stages in my discussions so far.

It's possible that our first reaction to Scadding's argument will be broad agreement. In reacting this way, we will be thinking, perhaps, of earlier reading and study on health and disease, which has identified and privileged objectivist conceptions of these things. We may also be thinking back to aspects of our professional experience. The nurse, say, will be recalling ward reports; the litany of disease they conveyed and the lines of beds of incapacitated patients that were passed as the report was given. The radiographer will remember the sallow person whose X-ray revealed a large black mass on their liver. The physiotherapist will recall the elderly person with osteoporosis who struggled to reach his Zimmer frame. All these kinds of thoughts seem to match with Scadding's conception of disease and health:

> If someone asks, 'Am I healthy?', all the doctor can do is to seek for evidences of known diseases and for significant deviations of structure and function from expected norms and reassure the enquirer if he finds none. (Scadding, 1988: 123)

So his conception seems to match not only dominating conceptual and theoretical accounts of 'health' but also our practical experience. Yet if we allow ourselves space and distance for the purpose of reflection, it might be possible for us to do two kinds of things:

▸ We might be able to recognise that what moves us towards a Scadding-like position on health are our beliefs and values, which have been shaped by our theoretical encounters and our professional experiences. We are not moving towards that position on the basis of fact and description alone (Hare, 1986).

▸ We might then in turn move from dominant conceptions (health is *the same as* disease absence) to alternative ones. For example, we could allow ourselves the time to think about theory that puts interpretivism, rather than objectivism, in the foreground (e.g., Seedhouse, 1986, 2001). Or we could think about the idea of health as a social or public creation rather than an individual responsibility or misfortune (Wilson, 1976; Cribb, 1982). These are real possibilities for us to uncover if we allow ourselves the opportunity to analyse our experiences, relating them to other aspects of our understanding in an inclusive, 'whole person' way.

Towards New Ways of Understanding and Behaving

This takes us to the next stage of a reflective learning cycle. From analysis of the experience, we move to new understanding and so (potentially at least) to new ways of behaving, thinking and feeling (Boud, Keogh and Walker, 1985). New, altered understanding seems to be a self-evident product of genuine reflective analysis. The nurse, say, who turns from ward reports to interpretive accounts of 'health' may well eventually change his understandings of the concept. But even if he continues to regard objective notions related to 'absence of disease' as the most reliable conceptual account (there is immense power, after all, in the daily experience of seeing diseased and therefore 'unhealthy' people), his understanding will still have changed. It will have done so because he will have engaged in evaluation of alternative conceptions and accounts; and because he will have examined the roots to the beliefs and values that govern his thoughts, feelings and actions connected to the idea of 'health'.

And there is at least the potential (and hope) that *changed understanding will lead to changed behaviour*. In a world which was always ideal, reflective learners – practitioners would always be able to use their new understanding to alter their behaviour. But both learning and practice contexts hold restrictions and limitations (Marshall and Rowland, 1998; Tate and Sills, 2004). We might wish to learn or practice in different ways, and reflection provides us with the 'evidence' that we need to do so, but there will always be limitations on our ability to actually accomplish this; things like time, policy direction, organisational support, resources and so on.

Given this, it may be best to talk about a *commitment* to change stemming from reflection, rather than a narrow *requirement* for us to do so. Sometimes – perhaps often – change just won't be possible. What is essential is that critically reflective processes allow at least the 'imagining and exploring [of] alternatives' (Clouder, 2004: 101). We should be able to do this by ourselves and hopefully with others. We may be able to enact those alternatives. It's possible that we won't. The important thing is commitment to a reflective cycle through which those alternatives become apparent as a result of our evaluations and re-evaluations. In this sense, the stage we have reached in the cycle of new understanding and potential change should only serve to lead us back to further experience and reflection.

Thinking Point

What obstacles can you identify in your own situation that would prevent you from engaging in change (either practice – or learning – related, or both) where the need for change seems to be a result of engaging in critical reflection?

Engaging in Reflection

From this account of reflection-on-action, we can identify two crucial requirements for engaging properly with the process:

▶ We need *a clear account* of the experience we're reflecting on;
▶ We need to find *ways of making sense* of it and opportunities for doing so.

The account of the experience provides the raw material for analysis. What actually happened? What was being thought and felt? How, though, do we produce this account? Educators tend to agree that it's done through *writing* about what happened (Tate and Sills, 2004). Even the best memories are inadequate, so students of health and health care need to keep a reflective diary (Tate, 2004). Some health professional-related courses encourage or require students to complete and submit reflective diary sheets (White, 2004). But there is a need to draw another distinction here:

- Between reflective *diary-keeping* on the one hand;
- And reflective *writing* on the other.

Diary keeping is the written recording of significant or memorable experiences as soon as possible after they've actually happened. Of course, diary-keeping will involve elements of reflective writing. For example, as well as describing the experience in terms of the action that took place, if it is going to be useful it will also ask (and perhaps begin to answer) evaluative – that's to say, reflective – questions. These might include:

- How did the experience feel?
- What was good or bad about it?
- What can be learnt from it?
- Could anything have been done differently? (White, 2004: 30).

Reflective writing stems from this initial use of these kinds of questions. They will stimulate thought and reaction that will, hopefully, make us want to add to our initial diary-writing-to say more about what we thought and felt and hoped. Again, health professional-related courses frequently require this kind of writing from students. Moreover, a number of health professions (e.g., nursing) demand evidence of reflection on practice demonstrated through reflective writing both to gain entry to the profession; and to maintain registration status (Barker, 2004). The requirement might take the form of completion of professional portfolios, clinical learning journals and so on.

I understand the distinction between diary-keeping and reflective writing to lie in the fact that the latter is an activity carried out with less immediacy to the experience itself. So it provides more opportunity to construct a response to the experience and analyse it. In sum:

> *Reflective writing gives a chance for more systematic evaluation, involving and integrating theory and literature to enlarge understanding of what happened and why, as well as how things might be different.*

Another way of representing the difference between reflective diary-keeping and reflective writing is in terms of 'writing down' and 'writing up', both of which contribute to 'writing through' an issue (University of Auckland, 1993: 41). I 'write down' observations, thoughts, memories more or less as they happen or occur to me. I 'write up' more polished accounts and discussions (of a particular experience, say) at some point after I've had time to consider and connect it with other aspects of my experience.

▶ 'Writing down' is the more or less immediate written recording of experience, although it should begin to ask questions aimed at evaluating (reflecting on) that experience. 'Writing down' is the function of the reflective diary.

▶ 'Writing up' is the less immediate but more considered analysis of the experience using, importantly, what has been written down. It also integrates theoretical and other perspectives gathered in the intervening time to form a wider understanding of the experience being reflected on.

Identify an experience connected to your health studies-related learning. Try and write about it in the way that I have discussed. Begin by 'writing the experience down' then move to 'writing it up'. How did you move from one kind of writing to the other? If there were difficulties in doing so, what form did they take and how might you deal with them?

It may take you a while to complete the process of moving from 'writing down' to 'writing up', so try and keep a record of what's going on in your writing, and your thoughts about the process.

Diary-keeping (or 'writing down') and reflective writing (or 'writing up') support each other's development. Health Studies students frequently find difficulty in engaging in reflective writing, which after all is a particular skill (Clouder, 2004). I argue that the more material, the more 'prompts' if you like that students have to work on, the greater is the chance of successful reflective writing. 'Writing down' helps to provide that material, especially if it starts to try and evaluate the experience – maybe by using some of the kinds of questions I suggested earlier. Generally speaking, it's possible to suggest that 'writing [an experience] down' (description and perception) is perhaps a less rigorous task than 'writing it up' (analysis of the experience and trying to relate it to wider contexts and understanding). 'Writing down' can provide a helpful bridge between our experience and any requirement to offer a formal written reflection on it (a requirement that may be summatively assessed).

Despite this account, it's probably still reasonable for somebody to ask, 'Yes, but what do I actually *have to do* to write reflectively? At this point, I want to emphasise the importance of *questions* as a stimulus to reflection through writing (Tate, 2004: 13). The sense of structure that might come through using an appropriate question framework will, I suggest, help to develop confidence that reflective writing is achievable. Among the kinds of questions that Tate suggests could be useful stimuli to reflection are these:

▸ What were your hopes for the outcome in the incident [being reflected on]?
▸ How were your hopes related to your own expectations?
▸ What are the sources in your life and work for your ideas and values?
▸ Are these ideas and values still appropriate for you at this stage of your life?
▸ Why do you continue to endorse and act upon these ideas and values? (Tate, 2004:13).

Some of these questions (and the others in Tate's longer list) are ones that it might be useful to start answering as part of the process of 'writing down', the more or less immediate recording of experience (e.g., the questions on hopes and expectations). Responses to others may need greater time to germinate and could emerge in part through the more measured and distant process of 'writing up'. All of the questions could have value right through the 'writing down' to 'writing up' process.

I want to move now to the second crucial requirement for engaging properly in reflection. This is the need to find ways of making sense of the experience, and opportunities for doing so. It should be clear that the process of writing itself and the opportunities for critical self-examination it ought to allow us present opportunities for sense-making. Our engagement in writing, along the lines that I have described it, moves us from just an account of what happened to detailed analytic and reflective understanding of why we thought, felt and acted in the way we did.

For some people, reflective writing is sense-making enough in itself. It's all that they want, or need, to do. But for others, the process of making sense of things will extend beyond the individual act of writing.

It might involve benefiting from the insights, perceptions, comments and questions of others, with the aim of achieving more rounded understanding. There are good reasons for listening to others. While we all enter into self-examination with a commitment to honesty in the resulting reflections, having the touchstone of others' insights is a way of maintaining balance and rigour. It's perhaps natural for us sometimes to find it difficult to challenge ourselves. We may become unduly negative about who we are and what we do; or we may engage in self-deception (Tate, 2004). Supportive exchange with others can help avoid these things.

In truth, worthwhile critical reflection probably very often requires investigating both ourselves and seeking the thoughts of others; we need both *monological* and *dialogical* reflection (Habermas, 1972):

▶ *Monological* reflection involves developing a 'dialogue' with ourselves. Methods might include portfolio development, diary and essay writing.
▶ *Dialogical* reflection involves developing a dialogue with others. Methods might include role-play, simulations, tutorials and web-based discussion forums (Clouder, 2004).

These and others are all methods that might be used in health studies-related teaching and learning to encourage reflection and develop reflective capacity. Indeed, engaging in some or all of them is likely to be a *requirement* for many health studies students. Each method might have certain features:

▶ It might be *supervised* (e.g., reflection-centred seminars); or it might be *unsupervised* (say, peer support groups):
▶ It might be *assessed* (either formatively or summatively), or it might not be subject to assessment at all.
▶ It might take place in a *formal* setting (such as an academic institution) or it might take place very *informally*.

Thinking Point

Thinking about *how* you might engage in reflection has prompted me to draw a number of distinctions:

▶ Between *monological* and *dialogical* reflection;
▶ Between *supervised* and *unsupervised* reflection;

Thinking Point *continued*

▸ Between reflection that is *assessed* in some way and that which isn't;

▸ Between reflection that takes place in a *formal* setting and that which takes place *informally*.

Consider the opportunities for reflection that you are presented with. Using the distinctions that I have drawn, try and establish their nature. Are you presented with a range of different opportunities? It might be helpful to think about your reaction to each kind of opportunity. What are its strengths and weaknesses? What sort of reflective opportunity do you find most – and least – helpful? Is there a way of increasing the kinds of opportunities for reflection that you personally find the most helpful?

Critical Reflection and Health Studies: Adding to the 'Rough Guide'

In the same way that I did at the end of the previous chapter on critical analysis and health studies, I want now to offer my 'rough guide' to using critical reflection as a way of understanding the field and its complexities. My argument has been that we need both critical analysis and critical reflection to help our understanding. So the summary of stages in critical reflection that I'm now setting out needs to be used together with the summary I offered at the end of the last chapter. And we need to remind ourselves again that the process of critical analysis on the one hand, and of critical reflection on the other, are strongly connected to each other.

Stages in Critical Reflection on Health

Stage 1: Plotting the Connection between Critical Analysis and Critical Reflection

Confronted with an experience in practice or learning (a particular health-related argument, say), it's possible to consider the argument reasonable but still not be convinced by it. Why is this so? One answer to this question is to recognise the limits of rational argument in the field of health studies and the importance of

Stages in Critical Reflection on Health   *continued*

beliefs and values in determining our positions. We need generally to recognise the nature of critical analysis and critical reflection and how they connect to each other. In particular contexts, we should try to identify the *limits* of analysis and begin to imagine how *reflection* might also help us in understanding our confusion or our ambivalent reactions.

Stage 2: Understand Yourself as Engaged in 'Whole Person Learning'

If analysis by itself is not sufficient to understand a health studies-related experience, we need to extend beyond it. We also need to understand the connection between practice and theory, and the nature of learning in relation to both, in order to make sense of our field. This means that we are engaged in 'whole person learning', which might be quite different from the kind of teaching and learning we have previously been used to.

Stage 3: Avoid Intimidation!

Critical reflection is often represented as a complex process. There are good reasons for this; conscientiously undertaken, reflection demands care and commitment. But we need to temper this with the idea that we employ reflection in our daily lives and decision-making.

Stage 4: Build Up an Awareness and Understanding of Models of Reflection

The complexity of reflection, of how thoughts, ideas, emotions and feelings work on each other, is daunting. But it can be helped by the use of appropriate models. I have used one particularly in this chapter, but there are others. Explore the others that are available, using the references I've cited in this chapter. Find one that makes sense to you, and helps you in understanding complexities. But remember that models, while they're helpful, are only representations of a much more involved reality.

Stage 5: Reflect on the Experience

Preparing as I've suggested in the previous stages should make it easier for you to engage in reflection itself:

▸ Make yourself open to experience;
▸ Take time to record it in writing;

Stages in Critical Reflection on Health   *continued*

▸ Use questions to help structure your reflective writing, or writing that will support reflection ('writing down' and 'writing up');

▸ Develop an awareness of your preferences for how you reflect, while generally recognising that both reflecting on your own and reflecting in ways that allow you to gain the insight of others are both useful;

▸ Be aware of (and maybe try to create more) opportunities for reflection, especially those that match your reflective preferences.

Turning Point?

In this chapter as well as in earlier ones, I've discussed the importance placed by professional education and training policy on critical reflection. It is an expectation that those wanting to train and enter a profession become competent critical reflectors. The rationale for this is in turn tied to wider health and health care policy. Competence or expertise in critical reflection will lead to changed and more effective learning and practice. Effectiveness and efficiency in health care are the by-words in current government policy, manifested through such processes as clinical governance (Scally and Donaldson, 1998).

We may well agree with all this. However, there is also the need to consider the possibility that reflection presents difficulties. I want to use this Turning Point to encourage thinking about the potential for conflict between the idea of reflection on the one hand, and health-related public policy on the other.

Reflection, as I've discussed, is a process that requires time. It also implies trust, particularly where there is exposure to the views of others either informally or formally (through, for example, assessment) (Tate and Sills, 2004). In the current context of both learning and health care, the drive for effectiveness and efficiency may make the time required for proper reflection difficult to come by. It may also make genuine trust harder to achieve as educators and managers strive to move in the particular directions demanded by

Turning Point? *continued*

policy – directions which might be incompatible with the beliefs and values of individual students and professionals.

A key difficulty also emerges in contemplating the relationship between reflection and change. The central purpose of reflection is the identification, through deep contemplation of experience, of new ways of thinking and behaving. But what if these new ways fail to conform to the expectations of those supervising the learner or managing the professional? It is clear that those in charge of policy and practice have certain expectations and agendas. What if these are challenged through reflective processes? This is not so unlikely. Freire's (1972) process of conscientisation (consciousness-raising), used to radicalise the urban poor of South America can be regarded as one forerunner of current notions of reflection.

The dilemma is this. If processes of critical reflection are allowed free rein, then we will be engaging in genuine reflection but we may end up in positions of conflict with those managing or supervising us. If reflection is in some way 'controlled' for outcomes that are deemed suitable, then it can't really be seen as reflection at all. To what extent, then, do you think that genuine critical reflection, the process I've tried to discuss in this chapter, is possible in current educational and professional contexts?

What's gone on in this chapter?

I've justified the importance of a focus on critical reflection for the health studies student, allied with one on critical analysis. Developing capacity in relation to both will help us understand the nature of health-related argument at both its 'rational' and its 'emotive' levels. I've discussed ways in which it might be possible to engage in reflection, paying particular attention to the idea that *writing* supports reflective processes. There is a range of ways through which it is possible to develop reflection and reflective capacity, and sustain 'dialogues with yourself', as well as dialogues with others. There is a need to think carefully about how you can take part in such processes, as well as what limitations structures and organisations might place on your ability to reflect (and perhaps more importantly to change practice as a result of reflection).

Part III
Critical Perspectives
on Health

7 The Nature of Health: Critical Perspectives from Philosophy

What is this chapter going to do?

In the final part of this book, I take the lessons of its first two parts about the nature of 'the difficulty of health studies', and the processes required to make sense of this difficulty. I apply what has been learnt to a small number of academic disciplines (or sub-disciplines) in order to try and understand, as well as critique, some of their 'critical perspectives on health'. Each of these disciplines (or sub-disciplines) claims to tell us something important about health. In this chapter, I am going to consider the possible contribution of philosophy to understanding the *nature* of health. The illumination philosophy might especially provide comes as a result of its concern with *conceptual* enquiry – and in particular concepts that are subject to dispute and contest. Through the use of philosophical conceptual enquiry, it seems possible to establish that 'health' is not the same kind of concept as 'disease'. So 'health' can't be simply 'disease absence'. Philosophy suggests to us that in developing an understanding of health, much depends on how we talk about it. Our talk creates the context for our understanding of the concept, so we need to analyse carefully how and why we engage in the talk that we do about health.

Critical Perspectives: A Return to Ontology

In this chapter I am going to return to one of my earliest themes, which first emerged towards the beginning of Chapter 1 and has since appeared at various points in my discussion about 'the difficulty of health studies'. It is the question of the nature of health.

This question is an ontological one; that is to say, it concerns the nature of the existence of something. Ontological questions are a central part of metaphysics, one of the main branches of the discipline of philosophy (Lacey, 1976). So I'm seeking the help of philosophy as I consider again questions about the nature of health. What *is* this nature? Why do we consider it has such a nature? How can we justify and defend our views? With the benefit of our explorations on the processes of critical analysis and reflection, I hope that philosophy can supply us with grounds for critical perspectives on the nature of health. It's also possible that analysis and reflection will help us to become clearer about what philosophy is actually offering us. In other words, the project in this chapter (and this final part overall of the book) has the potential to work in two different ways:

▸ It could help us to see what insights on 'health' philosophy (and in the following chapters, other subject areas) can provide us with;
▸ And it could help us evaluate the worth of those insights.

The Nature of Philosophy and its Connection to the Study of Health

One of the embarrassing difficulties faced by the professional philosopher is that she may find it hard to define what her profession involves:

'What is philosophy?' is itself a philosophical question. (Lacey, 1976: 159)

But to save time, I'm going to take the risk of offering some kind of definition! We can define and describe it in two ways:

▸ According to its *subject matter;*
▸ According to the *methods* that it uses (Lacey, 1976:159).

Both ways will be useful in understanding why we are using philosophy to try and gain a critical purchase on the nature of health.

The Subject Matter of Philosophy

Philosophy can be seen as having three main subject branches: metaphysics, epistemology and ethics.

▸ *Metaphysics* is the study of the nature of being, or existence. The concerns of metaphysics and the ontological questions (questions related to being) it has posed have traditionally been wide-ranging.

They are the kinds of questions that we might naturally associate with philosophers (at least the wild-haired, untidily dressed, ivory tower-inhabiting caricatures of our imagination!). What is time? What is space? What kind of a being is God? What does it mean to be a person? But we can ask questions about the nature of being and existence of anything (Lacey, 1976) and in this case we are asking them about the nature of health.

▸ *Epistemology* is enquiry into the nature and grounds of belief, experience and knowledge (Duncan, 2001). What can we know about something? How can we know it? These are important philosophical questions and ones that are relevant to the study of health, as I argued at the very beginning of this book. I also argued that the connection between ontological and epistemological positions on 'health' is close and reciprocal. Depending on our beliefs about the nature of health (what kind of being it has), we will formulate certain beliefs about the knowledge that we can have of it. If I believe, say, that health is 'the absence of disease', I'm likely also to believe that health (non-disease) is something which can be objectively measured.

▸ *Ethics*, on one view, is enquiry into how we ought to act and conduct ourselves (Duncan, 2001). Another view is that it concerns values and the assessment of what is valuable. I regard ethics as involving both questions of *action and conduct*, and questions of *value*. Once again, our thoughts about the nature of health and what we can know about it are likely to lead us to certain beliefs about the *value* of health. If I believe that health is 'the absence of disease', I will value health *because* it involves disease absence. (And from this will flow a whole range of values connected with how we ought to live our lives and how we ought to work in health care.)

The Methods of Philosophy

Generally speaking, what philosophers in all three branches of the discipline are doing is engaging in *conceptual* exploration. This is the basis of their methods, but what exactly does it mean?

Having a concept of something is being able to think and reason about that thing, whatever it is, and to be able to distinguish it from other things (Lacey, 1976). So philosophers are trying to establish how we think and talk about a thing, A, and why it is that we think and talk about it in that way. Given the importance of health, philosophical enquiry ought to have a natural concern with how we talk about the *concept* of health. Further, from my understanding of the nature of a concept, philosophers are also likely to be interested in whether thing A can be distinguished from concepts very often closely associated with it, and if so how and why? What is it that makes A, say, different from B? So in the field of health studies, then, we might expect philosophy to help us, for example, with an investigation into whether, how and why the concept of 'health' differs from the concept of 'disease'.

Philosophy concerns itself especially with what I've previously called *contested* concepts. One of the central components of my argument for 'the difficulty of health studies' was the disputability and contestability of health itself. Given this, we may be able to use philosophy and its natural inclinations to careful conceptual enquiry to help us move closer to a proper understanding of the nature of health.

If we are involved in conceptual enquiry, in trying to establish how we think about something and how it differs from other things we think about, then our methods must be *analytic*. We must be prepared to examine the concept of concern to us, to break it down into its constituent parts so that we begin to get a clearer picture of what its nature is. But this analysis is of a particular kind. In dealing with contested concepts – in this case health – we are trying to understand how and why people talk about something whose nature is fundamentally disagreed upon. This disagreement has arisen at least partly because we can't point to something in the empirical world and say, 'Look, just look at that. *That's* what health is.' It's true, as we've seen, that one version of an objectivist account of health is to argue that it's the absence of disease, when disease is something that at least to some degree we can in fact point to. But this account is nowhere near as straightforward as the 'Look at this, that's what it is' kind. As I'll discuss shortly, the objectivist argument involves highly problematic additional assumptions.

We dispute the nature of health because there is no *material referent* we can agree on-something existing in the real world that definitely represents the concept we are talking about. Because there is no indisputable material referent related to the concept, we talk about it in different ways. There is no definitive empirical discovery to be made. Instead we are analysing decisions people have taken on how they talk about a given concept (Sprague, 1978). Here we are analysing the decisions people make about how they talk about the concept of health.

At this point, some people may well feel frustration. If we can't see it, they might say, what's the point of trying to pretend we can analyse and understand it? What's the use of philosophical conceptual enquiry? We might as well just take a straightforward account (health as the absence of disease, for instance) and do our best to work with that. What's the use in trying to do anything else?

Thinking Point

What is the use of philosophical conceptual enquiry into the nature of health? From the accounts I've built up of the 'difficulty of health studies' and methods of dealing with this (through critical analysis and critical reflection), try to develop your own argument for the value of philosophical conceptual enquiry in the field of health studies. Alternatively, if you find it hard to see value, try to develop an argument against conceptual enquiry.

Try to develop your argument (whether it's for or against) before you move on from this Thinking Point.

Trying to develop your own defence (or critique) of philosophical conceptual enquiry as it might be applied to health and health studies is important. It's important not least because, as with all other careful study in our field, it entails costs of time and energy. My own view is that this kind of enquiry into fundamentally disputed concepts is essential. Why?

▸ There are actually lots of concepts that we find out more about 'only by learning what to say about them' (Sprague, 1978:10). (And by implication, we can therefore only understand them by learning how and why people speak as they do.) These include, I think, concepts such as love, freedom and humanity – as well as health, of course. If we neglect examination and discussion of such concepts, we will be missing out much in terms of understanding our world, others and ourselves;

▸ One of my key claims in this book has been that our problems in studying health relate not only to conflicting arguments within the field but also to the differing values, beliefs and ideologies that more often than not underlie these. In trying to examine how and why people speak as they do about the concept of health, we should extend beyond critical analysis of their talk and their supposedly rational argument. We should also encounter and be able to examine the values from which their arguments stem. Moreover, it might be possible (as I'll discuss in Chapter 8) to reflect on how and why our own values and our own talk match with (or differ from) the talk and the underlying values of others. In this way, philosophical, conceptual analysis ought to move us towards a more complete analytic and reflective understanding of the nature of health.

The Trouble with Health Objectivism

I've been troubled by the arguments of the health objectivist from the very beginning of this book. There seems to me to be something fundamentally wrong with the claims of an objectivist such as JG Scadding, who I've taken as representative of the health objectivist's position. (The health objectivist is someone who takes the view that we can objectively define and describe an entity that we call 'health'.) Here is the nub of Scadding's argument again:

> If someone asks, 'Am I healthy?', all the doctor can do is to seek for evidences of known diseases and for significant deviations of structure and function from expected norms and reassure the enquirer if he finds none. (Scadding, 1988: 123)

We can point to abnormality of structure and function and call it 'disease'; we can do no more, in talking of 'health', than point to normal structure and function. So 'health' can be nothing other than the 'absence of disease'. There's no doubt that the clarity of this argument might appeal to some people. So why am I doubtful about it? There are two key reasons:

▸ First, other more interpretivist accounts of health (e.g., Seedhouse, 1986, 2001; Downie, Tannahill and Tannahill, 1996) have struck me as being fairly plausible. This plausibility, combined with a view that there is certainly *some* sense in connecting 'health' to 'disease absence', has moved me towards my position at the moment – health seems to be a genuinely contested concept (Gallie, 1956).

▸ Second, though, a straightforward objectivist account seems rather out of place in the complex territory of health studies, in which beliefs and values (especially professional beliefs and values) play such an important part. The simplicity of the objectivist account is momentarily soothing, until we're plunged back into the ideology and value-ridden territory of our field.

Now with the use of the insights and techniques of philosophy, I want to argue that the health objectivist is making a fundamental mistake:

The objectivist is making the mistake of believing that health is the same kind of concept *as disease.*

If my argument that this is a mistake is accepted, it allows us to pay much more attention to the idea I've raised that our construction of the concept of health depends to a large extent on 'learning what to say about it'. We learn what to say about health largely as a result of being involved in particular and particularly influential personal and professional contexts (and it's through involvement in particular contexts that the health objectivist makes the mistake that he does about the nature of the concept of health). So:

Mistaken conceptual use emerges as a result of how we 'learn to speak about health', including where and when this learning takes place. This process of 'learning how to speak about health' requires careful thought.

Thinking Point

Consider the two ways I've outlined above for starting to understand 'the trouble with objectivism';

▸ 'Health' is not the same kind of concept as 'disease';
▸ We need to pay much more attention than objectivism allows to how and where we learn to say what we do about it.

Which of these two ways would be best suited to being explored through a critically analytic approach? And which is best suited to a critically reflective approach? Or do we need to employ both approaches for each way?

Health is Not the Same Kind of Concept as Disease

I argue that this route to understanding the trouble with objectivism depends largely on a critically analytic approach. It is about trying to disassemble and then examine ways in which we think about and use the concepts of health and disease. From this, it should be possible to determine whether they are the same kinds of concepts, and so whether the assertion that health is no more and no less than the absence of disease is true. If they are in fact the same sorts of concepts, then it might be reasonable to infer a straightforward relationship between them, which might allow for one to be characterised as the absence of the other. If not, then the relationship between the two concepts becomes more complex and wouldn't necessarily allow the objectivist's characterisation. For example, we can talk about 'dark' as the absence of light because both 'dark' and 'light' are the same kind of concepts (both are to do with levels of radiation produced by the sun). But we can't speak of 'dark' as the absence of rain (without seeming ambiguous or appearing to talk nonsense) because they are clearly not the same sort of concept. (While both are concepts of the natural sciences, one is to do with radiation and the other with the condensing of atmospheric moisture.)

This example in fact gives a clue to the difficulty faced by the objectivist trying to claim that 'health' and 'disease' are sufficiently alike in a conceptual sense to talk of the former being no more than the absence of the latter. In talking about 'light' and 'dark' in a scientific sense, we are thinking of the same principles of physics applied to both concepts. But when we talk about 'disease' and 'health', is there a similar commonality of principles that would warrant as close a connection? An objectivist like Scadding believes there is. He believes that it is possible to think and reason about disease using the principles of the methodological nominalist (that is to say, someone who believes that a concept can be defined and understood by relating words or other symbols to observable phenomena). So 'disease' and its whole vast terminology (from asthma to yellow fever) form the language (often very precisely, at least as far as physical conditions go) that we use to describe observable stages in the processes of diagnosis.

'Health', though, doesn't seem to be the same kind of concept as this at all. Unless we accept that it is simply the absence of diagnostic observations (which actually does no more than beg the question of whether health is disease absence), it's hard to see how the concept of health can be subject to the same sort of methodologically nominalist account as disease. What observable phenomena relate to health? How are they identified and described? We can clearly ask these questions about disease, but I want to claim that we can't ask them in the same way about health. If we were to try and talk about observable phenomena related to health, we would not naturally attempt precise description of physical structure or function – or at least this would be only part of the story we would want to tell. We'd want to talk also about things like:

- Health as something that helps us to *flourish* (Baelz, 1979);
- Health entailing the *correct relationship between man and environment;*
- Health supporting *the capacity to make what we can of our lives* (Wilson, 1975);
- Health involving broader ideas of *'well-being'* (Downie, 1990).

In fact, we may want to talk only about these kinds of things, in preference to narrow physical function. They are, of course, quite different kinds of characterisations to those involved in the tight, nominalist account of disease offered by the objectivist Scadding.

It could be argued that in drawing attention to the sorts of characterisations of 'health' that I have done, I'm simply expressing my own personal preference for broader, more interpretive accounts of the concept. This may be so, except that all I've done is to try and respond to the objectivist – nominalist's demand for description. I haven't been able to come up with a convincing enough account of health that relies on 'observable phenomena' alone. As a consequence, I've had to plunder a wider vocabulary, involving terms that seem much more diffuse and oblique. Perhaps the distinction that might be drawn between 'negative health' and 'positive health' (Downie, Tannahill and Tannahill, 1996) will help in mapping what is taking place here:

- *Negative health* can be characterised as freedom from the burden of disease. It is *perhaps* amenable to tight, nominalist classification to the extent that in part it entails the absence of the observable phenomena that form the basis of our understanding of 'disease'.
- *Positive health* involves a completely different range of classifications and characterizations – 'flourishing', 'well-being' and so on.

That it seems necessary to talk, at least partly, in these two different ways about 'health' is strong evidence for not believing it to be the same kind of concept as disease.

What we Understand by Health Depends on How we Learn to Talk About it

I want to move on now to think about how (as well as when and where) we learn to talk about 'health' in the ways that we do – ways that struggle with (or perhaps embrace) wider classifications beyond 'disease absence'. Doing this will move us further along the road towards understanding the trouble with health objectivism. It will require further analysis of the nature of concepts in general and how we work with and use them. But as an enquiry about *how* we learn conceptual use, it will also demand a degree of reflection.

Thinking Point

Reflect on your current conceptualisations of 'health'. What experiences have shaped your thoughts about its nature?

Let's return for a moment to Sprague's argument for the class of concepts (and he argues there are many within this class) that are found 'only by learning what to say about them' (Sprague, 1978: 10). What exactly does he mean by this? In the first place, there is a need to point to the very large number of concepts that we can think about in a fairly straightforward kind of way. My concept of 'cake' or 'car' or 'mountain', say, will probably be much the same as yours – or at the very least, if we begin to argue about such things, we can probably fairly soon reach agreement or some kind of shared understanding. This is because these sorts of concepts possess what I've previously called 'material referents'. I can point, for example, to the smart Porsche at the top of the street and tell the person I'm arguing with that this is included in my concept of 'car'. Likewise, they can point to the battered Mini at the bottom of the street and suggest that this is included in their own conceptual understanding of 'car'. And we can probably agree that there is enough in common between the Mini and the Porsche to include both in what now becomes a shared conceptual understanding.

However, the class of concepts that we find out about 'only by learning what to say about them' is different. It includes apparently mundane things like sandwiches, and policemen. They might be mundane, but in each of these cases, unless we know how to talk about the thing concerned, we won't recognise it as such. If I didn't know how to talk about a sandwich (a combination of bread and filling), then I would see the food in front of me as simply that – two pieces of bread with something in between. I may think that I can easily point to a policeman as someone in a certain kind of uniform, but what about plain clothes detectives, or secret policemen, or policemen who are off-duty? (We would still expect these latter to act as policemen in an emergency.) Here again, we use the word 'policeman' because we have learned to talk about all these sorts of people in a particular way. We have collected them together and identified certain common features (e.g., the authority they all have) in ways that enable us to refer to each of them as 'a policeman'.

It could be argued that these examples are not so very different from that of the Porsche and the Mini I used just before. In the case of sandwiches and policemen, there are still material referents to which we can point and in doing so clear up misunderstandings about the concept concerned. ('Yes, it's true the man sitting in the corner of the bar isn't wearing a policeman's uniform, but I happen to know that he's carrying a detective's warrant card.') This is true to an extent. The difference, however, lies in the fact that the material referent (the man in the bar) is not enough in itself to convince the person I'm arguing with that the loner with the drink is a policeman. They need to know, as do I, about the various ways we can talk of 'policemen', which include policemen in plain clothes.

Now, though, Sprague moves to a rather more complex example. When I ask my bank manager for credit, to buy myself a new computer for instance, we are both able to understand what is being requested (credit) again only because we have learnt how to talk about it. If she gives me the credit, I can go out and spend the money, and to the assistant in the computer shop my cheque or my cash will simply be money, like any other kind. But to the bank manager and myself, it is money with a special status – it is credit *from* the bank, as well as a debt *upon* me. In this example, what appears as money to the assistant is not simply money to me (or to my bank manager). It is also an agreement, a commitment (on my part) and a signal of trust (from the bank manager). Credit is all of these things, yet we can only know it is all of them, and we can only understand it, if we know how to talk about it.

The example of 'credit' is interesting because while there are material referents that in some way relate to it, we cannot turn round, point to one of them and say, 'Look, *that's* credit!' The money I spend in the shop is the product of my agreement with the bank manager rather than the 'credit' itself. The letter she sends to me confirming the agreement is simply a letter and by itself would have no worth at all in the real world of the computer shop. The meaning of 'credit' – our conceptual understanding – lies beyond actual things; it lies within the way we talk and learn to talk.

I want to argue that 'health' is this kind of concept, one that depends on finding and learning ways to talk about it. As I've discussed, while there are a range of material referents that might in some way relate to 'health' (from 'disease' and its absence through to senses of 'well-being'), none of them can actually be said to *be* health itself. If this is the case, then meaning must lie in the way we talk about the concept. The fact that people talk about it in different ways (from 'absence of disease' to 'well-being') suggests strongly in turn that separate people (or groups of people) undergo different ways of *learning to talk* about the concept.

Thinking Point

Building on the previous thinking point, who or what has been influential in your own 'learning how to talk about health'?

I want to argue that we all learn how to talk about health from a number of different sources. These might include family, friends and school. Crucially, if we are health professionals, *we learn to talk about 'health' through our professional training and experiences and contacts*.

We will be learning through the litany of disease conveyed in the ward reports, the black mass in the liver X-ray, the frail elderly person with osteoporosis – the examples I suggested in the last chapter to represent the sorts of things shaping our professional understanding of 'health'. All these sorts of things will be important, and will remain so, in our own personal and professional 'learning to talk about health' because they are small representations of a much broader, deeper and ultimately dominating discourse on health. This is the discourse of Western biomedicine, which has moved us from ancient, Aristotelian concerns with the tripartite division of the human person into body, soul and mind (and thus 'health' constituting a 'unity of [these] parts in equilibrium' (Haldane, 1986: 147)). Biomedicine has moved us from thinking and talking of health in this unified, holistic way to conceptions that are both reductionist and focused on the idea of it being to do with 'normality' (Seedhouse, 1986, 2001). The shift has taken place not because 'health' itself has changed, at least in the sense of alteration to one particular material referent – such a thing doesn't exist. What has happened is that the way we speak, and the way we learn to speak, about the concept has altered. This changed way of speaking has been one of the products of the immense growth in status and power of just one of the many possible material referents to health – biomedicine.

Strengthening Health Interpretivism

Philosophical conceptual analysis, together with reflection, has led to the view that straightforward health objectivism ('health as the absence of disease') appears an untenable position. Two reasons for this view have been identified:

▸ There is no justification for regarding 'health' as sufficiently similar in a conceptual (or any other) sense to 'disease' to the extent that we can regard the presence of one as *the same as* the absence of the other. 'Health' might in part entail disease absence; but this absence cannot form a *sufficient* condition for the presence of health;

▸ If 'health' lacks a particular, undisputed material referent, then it can only be understood by working out how people talk about it, and how they learn to talk about it. For health professionals this will involve to a large degree understanding how they learn to talk about it *as professionals*.

Rejecting objectivism naturally moves us towards health interpretivism, the view that conceptual understanding and meaning relies on essentially subjective responses. Interpretivism, though, poses its own problems for rigorous philosophical conceptual analysis. Are we to allow, say, that health constitutes 'anything and everything'? Conceptualising in this kind of way seems rather sloppy and lackadaisical. It may also have potentially dangerous practical results.

If we allow that health could be anything we might want to claim for it, the risk is that highly dubious things start to appear on the list of what is to be regarded as 'health'. Some people, for example, might argue that a comprehensive programme of eugenics is part of what comprises 'health', because it is about developing fit and capable people. While many others would instinctively disagree with this view, not least on the basis that humanity shouldn't become a massive engineering project, there is no conceptual reason why the 'anything and everything' interpretivist should reject it. Of course this is an extreme example, but there are many others where we are likely to be anxious about the implications of this sort of interpretive position – such as the area of harmful lifestyle behaviours. Should we agree, for example, that binge drinking is part of what comprises 'health' because some people find it a pleasurable activity?

It seems as if the implications of health as 'anything and everything' are pushing us back in the direction of objectivism. We want (maybe we're almost obliged) to suggest that there are limits to what might count as 'health'. In an almost intuitive but still highly important way, we are inclined to agree with the sense in the view expressed by Downie and his colleagues that 'there are better and worse lifestyles' (Downie, Tannahill and Tannahill, 1996: 5). So there are certain practices and behaviours that are more or less likely to count as 'health'. However, it's now important to ask these questions:

▸ If there are (or should be) limits on the extent to which we can talk of 'health' so that this talk is reasonable and meaningful, what are those limits?
▸ And who sets them?

Thinking Point

What limits would you want to impose in thinking and talking about what counts as 'health'? *Why* would you want to impose those limits?

Different people will respond in different ways to these questions. For me, say, 'health' might in part be constituted by a faithful, single partner relationship. For someone else, 'health' is a succession of enjoyable one-night stands (Duncan, 2002). I regard smoking, and drinking beyond moderate limits as 'unhealthy'. To another person, both of these things are part of the embodiment of 'health'. In each case, we will all have good reasons for taking the view that we do about what health is. It's likely that I won't be able to change the promiscuous person's view, nor they mine. So we start to enter the territory of values again, and the content of the next chapter.

Before I finish this particular discussion, though, there is some further help that the ontologist might be able to offer. In the process of learning how to talk about things, what we are partly doing as I have said is trying to distinguish them from other things (Sprague, 1978). And in the case of things that we know only by learning how to talk about them (that's to say, where there's no material referent that will help us settle differences), we are doing something else as well. We are creating the *context* in which that thing, whatever it is, actually exists. In relation to certain sorts of concepts (e.g., metaphysical concepts such as 'space' and 'time') if it weren't for our context-setting talk, the thing wouldn't exist at all (Sprague, 1978: 18). One of the intriguing things about 'health', though, as I discussed at the very beginning of this book, is that there are lots of things we can actually point to and say, at the very least, that it has something to do with 'health'. (Doctors, hospitals and the NHS were a few of the things that I mentioned.) So while our talk and our efforts to conceptualise health are context-creating (because we can't point to something and say, 'Look, that's *definitely* health!'), that is not the whole story.

Existing alongside, and connected in some way to our conceptions of health, are these kinds of what we might call 'health-related phenomena'. There are, I want to argue, two kinds of contexts in operation:

▸ The material context that at least in some way is related to health (doctors, hospitals, the NHS and so on);
▸ The context created by our talk (how we choose to talk about 'health').

My argument is that part of the mistake the health objectivist makes is to assume that the *only* kind of context at work is the material one. So doctors and hospitals, the NHS and disease become the sole point of reference for talk about health, which of course is conceived of as the absence of disease.

The mistake is crucial, but easily made. If our professional backgrounds and experience are so influential in forming the ways that we choose to talk about health, as I've consistently argued, then we will be naturally inclined to refer to contexts that seem to support our choices about how we talk. In a sense, the mistake being made by the objectivist is to blend unwittingly the context of (professional) talk with what seems like (and to some extent is) the related material context. In that blending they become one, to the exclusion of everything else – including other ways that it might be possible to talk about health.

But there are lessons that can be learnt from the error:

▸ We need to engage much more fully with the 'missed context', the one that's established by our talk. We need to pay much more attention to the range of different ways in which people talk about health – crucially, lay people as well as (if not more than) professionals;

▸ In doing so, we should be able to recognise that there is not simply one kind of material context related to health – that of hospitals and disease. Others exist as well.

One of these other contexts is that of everyday life. In our daily life, for the most part quite unthinkingly, we rely on our bodily fitness and our emotional and psychological capability to carry us through the demands that are made of us and to meet the challenges that are placed in our way. When we are pressed, we might talk about this fitness and capability, this capacity to get on with things and possibly to move in the kinds of directions that are right for our own lives, as 'health' (Herzlich, 1973; Cox *et al.*, 1987; Blaxter 1990). These sorts of 'lay' views on the nature of health, briefly reviewed in Chapter 1, are to some extent matched by the interpretive theoretical accounts we have come across (e.g., Seedhouse, 1986, 2001; Downie, Tannahill and Tannahill, 1996).

In examining 'lay' conceptions and interpretive theory, it's possible that if we are seeking an overarching explanation of what health is within these, we might land on the idea that it is about *functioning* (Hare, 1986). If we possess health, then we are better able to function as individuals and in our social relations; if we don't, functioning will be much more difficult. It might even become impossible.

It's important to be clear that saying health is *about* functioning isn't the same as saying health *is* functioning. If we tried to suggest that the two were in fact the same, we would risk falling once again into the kind of trap to which I've argued the objectivist has succumbed. This is the trap of assuming that only a certain kind of context can be connected to health. Our mistaken belief now would be that *only* the context of everyday functioning counts in terms of understanding what health is.

Falling into this trap would in fact be very clumsy. It would be far clumsier than in the case of the objectivist wedded to the idea of health as the absence of disease. The objectivist has seen powerful, material contexts in which 'health' and 'disease absence' appear to mean the same sorts of things. It is an easy (although mistaken) step from this to assert that they are in fact the same thing. But saying that health *is* human functioning is a much more substantial (and much less forgivable) mistake. It is less forgivable because both logic and common sense tell us that human functioning cannot be narrowly confined and described. The kind of capacity that I need to function as a university lecturer will be different at least in some respects from, for example, the capacity to function required by my neighbour, who tends coppices and makes hurdles near the small village where I live. The notion of human functioning is so wide that in saying that 'health is human functioning', we would simply become hostages to fortune.

But while we clearly can't say that health *is* functioning, I think we can argue, based on the empirical and theoretical evidence I have referred to, that it is in some way *about* it. Adopting this looser description (health as somehow associated with human functioning) in fact strengthens an interpretivist position against attacks that there is sloppiness in the 'health is anything and everything' account – potentially the ultimate interpretivist position. It is strengthened because now health *can't* be anything and everything. It has in some way to be associated with proper human functioning.

Of course, the question at this point becomes this:

▸ What is proper human functioning and what isn't?

There are certainly some things that we can fairly easily divorce from the notion of proper functioning. These would include things like forced restrictions on freedom, attempts at coercion and so on. Generally speaking, our idea of what it is to be and function as a human involves freedom and a capacity for autonomy (Shweder *et al.*, 1997). So our ideas about what is in fact entailed by the idea of 'health' start to become at least partly circumscribed once we associate it with human functioning. Interpretivism, in the sense of 'health is anything and everything' starts to become much more reasonable.

Ethics and Interpretivism

This strengthened interpretive position doesn't solve all our problems in deciding on the nature of health. But it does move us forward in a number of ways:

▸ It gives us a real alternative to the objectivist. Accusations of conceptual sloppiness don't sound nearly so convincing now that we have pinned ourselves down to a relatively specific interpretivist position (health as associated with proper human functioning);
▸ It provides us with the possibility of some degree of common ground between the objectivist and the interpretivist.

This second point needs some more explanation. In Chapter 1, I discussed the likely difficulty in objectivist and interpretivist 'agreeing to differ' on the nature of health. Now, though, the chance of a small degree of reconciliation exists. The objectivist says, 'Health is the absence of disease'. The interpretivist who adopts the strengthened position that I've described replies, 'I believe that health is associated in some way with proper human functioning. Disease is very likely to inhibit functioning. So to some degree, health is indeed related to the absence of disease. But if we think about human functioning, the capacity to get on in the world and to meet challenges, we need much more than simply not to be suffering from disease. If health is associated with functioning, it has to entail a great deal extra and not simply be founded on the narrow claim you are making.' In this reply, the interpretivist is allowing a measure of credence to the objectivist as well as a good deal of weight to the 'common sense' view that 'health' extends beyond disease absence, and beyond its most obvious material referents in the real world – hospitals, doctors and so on.

But the challenge now becomes a genuinely ethical one. It is to establish the nature of an account of health that sets limits on what we can reasonably understand by our association of health with human functioning. However, the limits shouldn't be set in order to constrain our understanding of 'health'. They should be established instead so that we can be clear about the reasonable and legitimate extent of our health-related work. They should be a way of determining the purpose of this work and how we move towards meeting that purpose, in the context of our actual or potential professional positions, as well as our beliefs and values. After all, this is the reason why the study of health is important. In pursuing this clearer understanding of the purpose of health-related work, based on careful understanding of the nature of health itself, we need to develop and critique ethical perspectives.

Turning Point?

At the start of this chapter, I claimed that the project of using philosophy to gain critical perspectives on health had the potential to work in two different ways:

- It might enable us to see what insights with regard to the nature of health philosophy might provide us with;
- It might also enable us to evaluate the worth of those insights.

Turning Point? *continued*

The insights that a philosophical conceptual approach to 'the difficulty of health studies' might provide are now clearer. Such an approach has suggested that:

▸ 'Health' can't be the same as 'the absence of disease' because 'disease' and 'health' are very different concepts;

▸ A great deal depends on the idea that 'health' is how we learn to talk about it – our talk creates a context in which we understand what 'health' actually is;

▸ There is a need to try and understand that we talk in different ways, so creating different contexts. Crucially, we must recognise that the talk we have that is inspired by the 'material referent' of services to manage and treat disease needs to be balanced by other ways of talking and creating context (such as the talk that connects 'health' with everyday function).

But the question remains – even if we accept these insights, how useful is it to do so? What is its worth? I have tried to place emphasis in this chapter on the helpfulness of philosophy in understanding and dealing with 'the difficulty of health studies'. For example, I've suggested that recognising how and from where we create different contexts for our health-related talk might be a way of reconciling the differences between the interpretivist and the objectivist.

Equally, though, it might be possible to argue for an alternative 'spin' on the use of philosophy to health studies.

It might be suggested, for example, that the conceptual separation of 'health' and disease' represents a serious and possibly disastrous uncoupling. When we connect 'health' with 'disease', we are clearly not doing so in an arbitrary way. As I've agreed, there is good cause from the world of 'material referents' to do so. One possible practical impact of trying to establish a greater distance and a more profound difference between the two concepts is that we begin to devalue the material referents that provide a background for the notion of 'health as disease absence'. Returning to the distinction between 'negative' and 'positive' health, we might be moved towards a position in which efforts to work in favour of 'negative' health (to treat and prevent disease) become of less value to us than the promotion of 'positive' health.

Turning Point? *continued*

There are at least two problems with this position, if we arrive at it. First, despite our efforts at conceptual clarification, ideas about what exactly 'positive' health is and what can be done to maintain and improve it are still much less clear than those to do with 'negative' health. If, for example, 'well-being' is associated with positive health, what exactly is it and how can it be promoted (Seedhouse, 1995)? Second, the dissociation of 'health' from 'disease' (of 'negative' from 'positive' health) potentially belies the importance and worth of the human project of countering and dealing with disease.

This is only one possible conclusion of a more circumspect evaluation of the worth of the kind of philosophical conceptual examination of health that I've tried to undertake in this chapter. This 'Turning Point' asks you to consider it, as well as to try and frame your own evaluations, whether positive or otherwise, of the use of a philosophical conceptual approach to 'the difficulty of health studies'.

What's gone on in this chapter?

I have discussed in this chapter the potential contribution that the academic discipline of philosophy might make in understanding 'the difficulty of health studies'. Philosophy, through its concern with conceptual examination and how we talk about difficult and disputed things, seems to move us to a position in which it seems unreasonable to regard 'health' as no more than 'the absence of disease'. In thinking carefully about how we talk about health, we begin to recognise that inclination towards objectivist accounts of health stems from our professional backgrounds and our involvement with one of the 'material contexts' of 'health' – the context of disease treatment services. But we need to consider the other contexts of health-related talk, which move us towards a wider understanding of health as somehow being associated with human functioning. The questions now are how we should understand that association, how we should value it and how we should engage in health work that maximises human functioning and capacity. These are questions of ethics.

8 The Value of Health: Critical Perspectives from Ethics

What is this chapter going to do?

I am going to move now from an examination of philosophy's use in tackling the difficulties inherent within the study of health to the helpfulness (or otherwise) of its 'sub-discipline' – ethics. Ethics apparently offers us help in working out what is the nature of health as a value; and, related to this, establishing what obligations ought to guide the activities of those working for health. I move in my discussion to the idea that in both cases, considering ethics is useful to some degree to health studies students. But there are limits to this use. In particular, values-based accounts of health – health as a 'set of values' and health as a single, fundamental value – raise problems. These centre round difficulties in agreeing to the values proposed and in trying to enact them in practice. With regard to ethical projects of describing obligations that ought to guide the actions of health care workers, we are confronted with questions of why we should agree to particular sets of obligations. We are also faced with the problem of how it is possible to manage dispute in relation to what we are obliged to do in specific cases.

The Limits of Health and Health Work

We've established that health is much more than 'the absence of disease' and that in some way it can be associated with the notion of 'proper human functioning'. But what do we actually understand by this? We need yet again to try and establish meaning. But this kind of enquiry into meaning needs to take a different turn. Understanding health as associated with proper human functioning leads us into the territory of values. In asking what we understand by proper human functioning, we are not simply posing a technical question. We are also enquiring into the nature of the value of being human and of the values that are likely to support and express the value of humanity. Being human is not simply (*perhaps* not even importantly) about possessing a certain kind of anatomical structure and having the capacity for certain sorts of physiological functions. The conception I have of myself as a human extends well beyond the mechanical facts of my existence. It embraces the thoughts, feelings, emotions and attitudes I have about myself and about others, as well as the quality of my relationships and the sense I have of my purpose in being (Glover, 1999).

If we can better understand this extended conception of being human, we will be able to move towards a worthwhile picture of proper human functioning and, by association, of health itself. If I assert, for example, that being human involves being able not only to function physically but also to process thoughts, emotions and feelings, to have fulfilling relationships with other people and to have a clear view of my own life purpose, then this will constitute a conception of health. It is also likely to be a rich and full conception. But it is likely to be problematic as well, because the chances are that my conception of being human (and therefore of proper human functioning, and so of health) will be different from yours. And both our conceptions will probably be different again from someone else's.

Thinking Point

Consider your understanding of what it is to be human. Why do you think you have that understanding?

We now risk being swept back to a 'health is anything and everything' position, with all the problems this involves. To avoid this risk, there is a need to engage in a certain kind of argument. It is an argument that is not only about establishing the nature of the value of being human, and of what values are likely to give fullest expression to the value of humanity (and therefore, by association, health). It is also an argument that is about attempting to claim a certain value or set of values, which *should have precedence over* another value or set of values.

In other words, we are allocating priority to one value or values set over another and in doing so are engaging in arguments of ethics. As this priority allocation is happening, what we are also doing, effectively, is to assert that our conception of proper human functioning will lead us to regard certain kinds of work for health as more important than others. This is because they are more likely to lead to fulfilment of the central purpose of health work, which is to maintain and enhance proper human functioning, however we now understand it. In fact, we might do more than this. We might say that we would not engage in any work that doesn't seem to match up with 'our' value or set of values. So our discussion and argument will possibly lead to two things:

▶ We will set limits on our view of the nature of health as a value;
▶ We will therefore set limits on what we regard as reasonable work for health.

In doing this, we remove the risk of being swept back to 'health as anything and everything'. However, the question now is whether we can justify the limits that we will have set on both the value of health and on what is work for health. Can we justify our limited interpretations? Part of this chapter is about examining claims and arguments that have been made in support of setting limits to health interpretivism; arguments for seeing health and the purpose and nature of health work in a certain sort of way, possibly to the exclusion of other sorts of ways. My view is that overall there are difficulties with these interpretive ethical accounts of 'health'.

But it isn't enough simply to say that there are problems with these kinds of attempts to limit our conceptions of the value of health and health work. If we are working in health, we need guidance on how we should undertake this work. In part this is also a matter of ethics and towards the end of this chapter I will be examining ways in which the moral obligations of health care workers have been framed and whether it is reasonable to accept such obligations. So this chapter has two central purposes:

▶ To establish the worth of accounts of the nature of health *as a value;*
▶ To establish the worth of accounts of the kinds of *obligations* that health care workers have (or ought to have) in their work for health.

But before we move to this examination of values and of obligations, we need to construct an account of ethics that justifies our considering the critical perspectives on health that it offers.

Thinking Point

Do you think it is important to consider ethics in relation to health and health work? Construct a justification for your view, drawing on both critically analytic and critically reflective perspectives.

The Nature of Ethics

I offered a brief description of ethics, one of the three main branches of philosophy, in the previous chapter. Ethics, I suggested, was concerned with questions of conduct, and with questions of value (Lacey, 1976). We seek help from ethics hoping that

▸ It will provide us with guidance on generally speaking *how we ought to act;*
▸ It will provide us with guidance on *what is valuable, or desirable.*

These two views of the purpose of ethics might sound relatively indistinct from each other. However, they represent two quite different ways of thinking ethically and two opposing ethical traditions. It's possible for someone to believe that consideration of how we act should precede any question of the value that might accrue as a result of the action. More exactly, value actually lies in always undertaking *that kind of action* rather than in say the consequences of the action.

To give an example, I might believe that I should always tell the truth, regardless of whether in doing so my truth-telling results in some kind of valuable or desirable outcome. We all know that in health care as well as in the wider world, there are occasions where truth-telling results in difficulties. The wife who long ago had an affair with another man; the 28-year-old woman about to get married who underwent an abortion at the age of 16; the doctor faced with the terminally ill patient who has given every sign that he doesn't want honesty about his condition. In all these and many other cases, telling the truth would probably not result in valuable or desirable outcomes. But some ethical theorists would continue to argue that we should always tell the truth (or keep promises, or pay our debts, or whatever it happens to be). Such theorists subscribe to *deontological* views of ethics:

▸ *Deontology* is the ethical view that there are some obligations that we have and need to undertake, regardless of the value of the associated probable outcome in doing so.

The father figure of deontological ethics is frequently seen as Immanuel Kant, the eighteenth-century German philosopher (1724–1804). Kant constructed a theory of ethics based on the fundamental importance of understanding human beings as rational. We are governed, Kant claims, by a reality independent of our everyday experience. The evidence for this, he argues lies in our being able to exercise our own free will, to have the capacity to act morally or otherwise, and not be subject to apparently random and capricious laws of nature. *Reason* exists independently of reality, and it is reason that moves us to act morally, out of duty for its own sake and aside from any consideration of consequences:

> I ought never to act in such a way that *I can also will that my maxim should become a universal law.* (Paton, 1948: 12)

This is Kant's first formulation, in his 'Groundwork of the Metaphysics of Morals', of what has become known as the categorical imperative. If my actions are to be moral, they must be performed out of duty, because otherwise they would not be based on reason, the independent reality that governs the actions of rational beings. I can't tell the truth, or keep promises, or pay my debts only sometimes and not others because if I did so, the world of human relationships and transactions would become chaotic and unmanageable. It would be reduced to the unpredictability of the natural world. Morality would collapse; indeed, it wouldn't exist at all.

Thinking Point

'I must act according to the duties or obligations that I have, independently of any consideration of consequences that might occur as a result of my dutiful actions.' What are the weaknesses in this ethical formulation?

It is important to remember that Kant was a philosopher of the Enlightenment. This is the eighteenth-century project we have discussed at various points in this book, and which was essentially founded on the belief that rational science could offer a total explanation of the human world and provide us with all the means necessary to develop ourselves. Given this context, Kant's own project of attempting to place reason and rationality at the heart of morality becomes more understandable. If intellectual understanding is being driven by a belief that the physical sciences can explain and deal with all, then why not apply this belief in the power of rationality to ethics? As with other areas of philosophical enquiry, Kant's argument is a conceptual one. More particularly, it is *a priori*. (Roughly, '*prior to* experience' and contrasting with an argument based on empirical evidence of some kind.) Kant can only *claim* that there exists a reality independent of experience, founded on reason. He can't actually *know* this, and so our conviction in his position rests on the strength of his argument.

Interestingly, Kant's conceptual, *a priori* argument for an 'independent moral reality' is rather different from the kind of conceptual arguments we were earlier trying to formulate and critique with regard to the idea of 'health'. In these, one of our starting points (and later on, touchstones) of argument was the idea that there are indeed things in the real world (doctors, hospitals and so on) that in some way represent certain conceptions of health. In fact, one of my conclusions towards the end of the last chapter was that the objectivist's 'mistake' in believing health is the absence of disease lies at least partly in their assumption that this material context of 'health' is the only one at work. Now though, in thinking about Kant's idea of an independent reality based on reason from which our moral obligations stem, we don't appear easily able to connect it to any material referent. At least, we can't do so in the way that it seems quite plausible to do so in relation to 'health'. We probably have an awareness of the concepts of 'reason' and 'obligation' (although understanding is likely to differ from one person to another), but what of an 'independent reality' founded on reason?

In itself, this isn't necessarily a problem. There are many *a priori* concepts and statements that we can more or less readily accept. I wouldn't quarrel, for example, with the concept of 'infinity', although this is logically *a priori*. (How can I experience infinity?) The difficulty with Kant's argument, however, is that aspects of our experience appear directly to contradict what he is asserting. The association between ethics and reason isn't mutually exclusive. We perhaps engage in something that we might want to call 'ethical reasoning', but this doesn't depend on reason (rationality) alone. When we 'reason' ethically, it is hard (probably impossible) to avoid contemplation of our feelings, emotions and reactions. All of these, as well as rational reason itself, are drawn into our deliberations. We talk quite easily of people being 'ruled by their heart rather than by their head', and don't necessarily think this is always a bad thing. Moreover, even if we do employ reason alone in our moral decision making (which is doubtful), this reasoning is unlikely to be devoted simply to working out which of my *obligations* should drive me in a moral sense. I will also think about the values that I hold as well as the consequences of what I'm thinking about doing and so on. Of course, there may be a correlation between all of these things. Then again, there may not be.

The point is that Kant's *a priori* argument in favour of reason and duty being at the centre of our moral compass seems to run in important ways directly against our ethical experience. We are not rejecting the argument on the grounds of it being *a priori* alone. Our doubts have emerged mainly because thinking about our experience in this area leads us to believe that an argument *'prior to* experience' is not going to provide us with a completely adequate account of ethics.

Difficulties with deontology move us for the moment from the idea of ethics providing us with guidance on how we ought generally to act towards the notion of it helping to establish what is valuable, or desirable. In particular, we need to consider the idea of consequentialist ethics:

▸ *Consequentialist* theory, as its name suggests, attempts to argue that what matters in our decisions about how we conduct ourselves are the consequences of our actions. Will they produce valuable or desirable results? The best-known consequentialist theory is probably *utilitarianism*.

The most famous advocate of utilitarianism is the ninteenth-century Scottish philosopher, John Stuart Mill (1806–1873). Mill's statement of the central principle of utilitarianism is appealing not least in its apparent clarity and simplicity:

> Utility, or the greatest happiness principle, holds that actions are right in proportion as they tend to promote happiness, wrong as they tend to produce the reverse of happiness. By happiness is intended pleasure, and the absence of pain; by unhappiness, pain, and the privation of pleasure. (Mill, 1962: 257)

According to this principle, thoughts about consequences and our intention that certain consequences should be produced (and others avoided) as a result of our actions represent prioritisation of our values. In acting, we aim to produce more of what for us is valuable and minimise the occurrence of the undesirable. The contrast with deontology is clear:

▸ The deontologist believes that what matters is that duty is performed and obligations are met, regardless of the consequences – the value lies in the performance of duty itself;

▸ The consequentialist utilitarian believes that action is only ethical if we perform it in the belief that it's going to produce the best possible consequences (the greatest happiness for the greatest number).

Thinking Point

'Action is only ethical if we perform it in the belief that it's going to produce the best possible consequences.' What problems exist with *this* formulation of ethics?

As with Kant and deontology, it's important to recognise Mill's utilitarianism as emerging from his own social times. The nineteenth-century was the period in which nations became more dependent on each other for trade and other reasons. It was also during this time that populations became increasingly inter-dependent. The Industrial Revolution prompted the development more strongly than ever before of towns and cities, of strangers coming together and having to rely on each other for services, employment and the general means to survive and thrive. Dependency of nation on nation and population on population led to the increasing importance of government. The need for an ethics that directed the conduct of government and others towards the best interests of the majority, in the context of the prevailing economic and social dependency, is clear.

But acting according to a belief that the consequences of the action will result in the production of what is valuable for most people means, of course, that there will be some that *won't* benefit. The government has decided, for example, that banning smoking in all public places will result in better health for most people. We may well want to support this policy. But there will be a minority (committed smokers with no intention of giving up) who will not benefit from the policy because they will be forced to relinquish the pleasure of smoking, say, in their local pub. Acting in the interests of the majority may well mean that the interests of the minority are not met. It may even lead to an inclination to play down or ignore minority interests.

A further criticism of consequentialist, utilitarian theory lies in the difficulty of the central idea itself – that our actions should be guided (and considered moral or otherwise) by thoughts about consequences. How can I ever *properly* know what are likely to be the consequences of my actions? I can sometimes predict these, and occasionally I might be quite certain in my predictions, but there are lots of times when I just won't know what's going to happen as a result of my doing something.

For the health care professional, this applies equally at the level of individual and population-based action. How does the doctor know that her advice on contraception will have positive consequences? Some of her patients may regard it as a licence for promiscuity and end up in a succession of damaging relationships, or suffering the effects of sexually transmitted disease. How does the administrator planning a population-wide cervical-screening programme know that the results will be entirely beneficial? There may be at least some people called to the programme who will be falsely identified as positive to testing and so suffer unnecessary psychological harm as they wait for confirmation of their diagnosis.

The point is that our actions can (and frequently do) have unintended or unexpected consequences. Some supporters of utilitarian theory have recognised the importance of this criticism and considered it so fundamental that they have tried to develop 'weaker' versions of the theory. In these, what becomes important is not the assessment of the likely consequences of individual actions; but rather the requirement to consider the consequences of breaking or keeping to certain action-governing *rules* (Urmson, 1967).

Thinking Point

Reflect on the two types of normative (action-guiding) ethical theories that have been considered – deontology and consequentialism. How useful do you think they are in understanding the problems of health and health care that we've been considering in this book?

Ethics Applied to Health Care

If the response to this Thinking Point is ambivalent, maybe pointing up doubt about the use of these ethical theories in our attempts to understand health and the purpose of health care, then this is understandable. The theories may well seem rather abstract and remote, despite my efforts to connect them to potential aspects of health and health care. A key challenge faced by present day ethics has been to try and offer a helpful response to the substantial anxieties faced by society over the nature of health care and shifting underpinning social conceptions of 'health' itself (Jonsen, 1998). This of course closely resembles the challenge of 'the difficulty of health studies' as I've represented it in this book. The responses offered by ethicists are frequently seen as being gathered together in one field, often labelled as 'bioethics':

> *Bioethics* is the systematic study of the moral dimensions – including moral vision, decisions, conduct and policies – of the life sciences and health care, employing a variety of ethical methodologies in an interdisciplinary setting. (Reich, 1995: 188)

This is a broad definition and its breadth is important for two reasons:

▸ It makes it clear that the territory of bioethics is not confined simply to medicine and medical practice. It is quite reasonable to use the 'methodologies' and techniques of bioethics to explore the particular questions we are trying to answer: what is the nature of the value of health, and of values that might be associated with health? In 'working for health', what moral obligations should we accept and employ in our professional lives?

▸ The implicit invitation within the definition to use a 'variety of ethical methodologies' in our exploration allows us to consider the worth of the ethical theories related to values and obligation that I have introduced (as well as adaptations by bioethics of these) in understanding difficulties connected to health studies.

The question now is how useful is bioethics in understanding and dealing with 'the difficulty of health studies'? It is a question that again needs a critically analytic and critically reflective response.

Values, Ethics and Health

The challenge accepted by some bioethicists is to argue that the value of health or values that are associated with health are so fundamentally important we face an essential *requirement* to work for 'more health'. Moreover, the nature of health as a value, or of values associated with it, dictate the way in which we should be involved in health work – they decide our purpose and our practice. We should be trying to achieve more of the value or values that are understood as being important.

If these kinds of arguments were convincing, they would have two important outcomes in terms of 'the difficulty of health studies':

▸ They would provide us with a distinctive agenda for our health-related work;
▸ They would help make much clearer the conception of health that was driving our work.

Given that the disputed and often vague understanding of 'health' that we often actually work with has been a major contributor to 'the difficulty of health studies', this second possible outcome seems especially useful. The question is whether bioethical arguments around the nature of the value of health are convincing enough. I want to consider two kinds of arguments related to the nature of the value of health:

▸ Argument centring around the idea that in thinking about 'health', we necessarily alight on a *set of values* that we must work towards maximising;
▸ Argument based on the idea that we can represent the value of health as a *single value*, the nature of which drives our work forward.

Thinking Point

Consider the idea that the purpose of our work should be about maximising what is valuable. In terms of the first kind of argument that I've mentioned (health as entailing a set of values) what would you want to include in that set? (You might consider including, for example, the value of disease absence, or the value of personal autonomy.) For the second argument (health as a single value) what for you would be the nature of this value?

A Set of Health-Related Values?

To begin with the first kind of argument – that work for health entails accepting a set of values and then trying to maximise them. Downie, Tannahill and Tannahill (1996) offer one such account. It is perhaps not surprising that after reviewing their interpretive account of health in the previous chapter (which like most realistic interpretive positions, tries to place limits on how we understand the concept), we now move on to assessing their account of the nature of values associated with health. Placing limits on interpretive positions ('health is this, but not this') necessarily implies attempts to justify the range of values associated with health and the nature of those values. (Or in the case of 'single value' accounts of health, to justify seeing the value of health in that particular way.)

Downie and his colleagues assert that there is a set of what they call 'necessary social values' (Downie, Tannahill and Tannahill, 1996: 158) that are closely associated with health, and which must be preserved and strengthened if health is to be maintained and improved. The values are necessary because they represent and respond to deep-seated human needs and nature.

For example, we know that human beings are vulnerable to disease, with all of the trauma, pain and discomfort that this brings. So we must commit to the value of physical integrity. This commitment would lead in turn to the value of avoiding unnecessary harm to others, in either a physical or psychological sense. We would probably want to formulate a moral principle to guide our actions so that they preserved and enhanced this value. Further values, such as respect for others' circumstances and convictions, motivate us towards additional moral principles. These include the need to work with benevolence and compassion, to try and advocate courses of action that will contribute to justice and fairness, and to have a concern for the best possible consequences for the greatest number of people as a result of what we do. In this way, the important connections between the values that we hold and the consequences that we seek are emphasised.

As well as necessary social values, Downie et al. also argue for the existence of a further set of 'necessary individual or personal values'. We need to recognise and uphold these values for ourselves (and others must encourage their development within us) so that we live worthwhile lives. The values are connected and cluster around a central notion of autonomy. They include self-determination, self-government, sense of responsibility and self-development (Downie, Tannahill and Tannahill, 1996: 167).

Crucially, necessary social and necessary personal values are closely linked. Neglecting one set or the other (or both) will lead to disharmony and possibly disintegration of society and self. Given this, it's now possible to see more clearly the kind of relationship that exists between the necessary social and personal values Downie and colleagues assert are connected with health, and health itself. If we don't hold these kinds of values and work to encourage their development, then health itself will falter and fail. Indeed, so close is the relationship that we could claim health itself as an embodiment of these values. If I have a strong sense of my own worth and direction, as well as that of others, in important respects I am properly healthy. In terms of Dworkin's (1995) classification of values, we could argue that the values are instrumental; we need them in order to survive and thrive in the world. However, they are also intrinsic because they embody what it is to be human itself and as such are irreducible to thoughts of their utility alone.

Thinking Point

Do you agree with Downie *et al.*'s list of necessary social and necessary personal values? If so, why? If not, for what reason-and what kinds of values would you want to put in their place?

If this kind of 'set of values' account is convincing it would, I've suggested, clarify our conception of health and so strengthen views of what our purpose is in doing health-related work. But the Thinking Point draws attention to a major difficulty in the argument of Downie and his colleagues. Why should we be prepared to accept the list of social and personal values that they propose as 'necessary'?

There are two reasons why we might be unprepared to accept some or all of these values:

▸ First, there is an implication within the argument that the two kinds of values, social and personal, automatically align with each other; that what is a good for our larger social context will also be good for us as individuals. But why should this be so? It's relatively easy to think of circumstances in which societal values clash with our own personal values and interests. For example, my value of self-determination might include a desire to take illegal drugs. I see this as positive (it alters my mood, expands my experience and so on.). Society, by definition, does not. Moreover, my individual drug-taking behaviour would quite possibly militate against the value of social justice. (I could quite likely become addicted to the drugs I was taking and ultimately need medical treatment and expensive rehabilitation, all of which would be putting an unfair burden on the state.)

▶ The second reason for being unprepared to accept these values is because of their general nature. They are essentially a set of liberal values, circling around the idea that we should be allowed to get on with our own autonomous lives and in general not interfere with the autonomous lives of others. Of course, liberal values are very important to many societies, especially Western democratic ones. However, they are not important to all societies. For some other societies, values might revolve instead around a general belief in *paternalism* (the idea that certain key figures in society know what is best for everybody else) or in *communitarianism*. (Values direct society members towards the good of the community overall rather than the interests and the freedoms of individuals.)

For those living in societies oriented towards values founded on principles other than liberalism, the difficulty is this. If the values proposed by Downie *et al.* come to resemble or take on the attributes of 'health' itself, as I've suggested might be so, they will allow far too much latitude with regard to what we see health as being. For example, the liberal might see smoking as contributing to individual health if it is freely undertaken and contributes to a sense of self-determination; it will stop being healthy at that point where it infringes on the autonomy of others. (Say, when non-smokers are subject to passive smoking in public places.) But the paternalist or the communitarian might well not allow smoking to constitute 'health' at all. The paternalist would argue that we know enough about smoking to assert that it damages the human body and causes disease; so society members must desist from the practice. The communitarian might argue that smoking causes diseases, smokers use health services much more than others and so they are failing in their responsibility to help create or maintain a just society. So their actions can't possibly be seen as 'healthy'.

If the values proposed by Downie and his colleagues are to be regarded as necessary contributors to health (even as health itself), then it seems very likely that at least some others will disagree with this assessment. This point is especially important given the multicultural context in which we frequently live – a context in which different people hold different understandings of which values are most important.

Health as a Single Value?

If we can't agree on a range of values such as those suggested by Downie *et al.* as being important to the maintenance and improvement of health, or even constituting health itself, is it possible to construct another kind of value-based understanding of the concept? Some bioethicists have argued that the proper way to understand health's value is to try and work out just one way of expressing such value.

From this single expression, they have argued that a range of further values (and associated moral principles) is likely to flow; together with the founding single conception of the value of health, they will provide us with sufficient direction in our health-related work. This is the kind of argument developed over a sustained period by David Seedhouse (see Seedhouse, 1986, 1988, 1997, 2001). We have encountered this argument earlier on, but now we need to consider it in our discussions about the worth of critical perspectives on health from ethics. Does Seedhouse's single value account (health as 'the foundations for achievement') help us to understand the concept of health better, along with what we need to do in order properly to work for health?

According to Seedhouse, health is what enables us to achieve our 'biological and chosen goals' (Seedhouse, 1986: 61). It follows, then, that our work for health ought to be about removing obstacles to the achievement of these goals. This 'negative' expression of the purpose of health work (it's about the removal of obstacles) is necessarily accompanied in Seedhouse's account by a 'positive' conception. We also have to value and work towards things that are likely to support its creation and improvement. So work for health should:

▸ Remove the obstacles to our goals;
▸ Create the conditions in which it will be easier to achieve our goals.

The nature of the distinction between Seedhouse's health as a single value argument and the multiple necessary personal and social values of Downie *et al.* should now appear clearer. In the single value argument, we accept the further values that flow from this value precisely because they emerge from it. Unless we agree in the first place with the idea of health as 'the foundations for achievement', we can't agree with the values that might flow from this conception (and therefore the nature of health work that needs to be done). For Downie and colleagues on the other hand, we must accept the multiple personal and social values they propose first (they are after all 'necessary') before we engage in work for health. Only if we do so will that work be adequate and appropriate.

So if we agree with Seedhouse that the single value of health is as 'the foundations for achievement', what does this suggest about the nature of the values that we accept contingent on this understanding? We might argue that these values include, for example, a commitment both to respect and to create autonomy (Seedhouse, 1988). If we respect autonomy, allowing people to make decisions about their own lives and futures, then we are not blocking the foundations for their achievement. On the other hand, if we try to limit autonomy, to intrude or coerce, then foundations will be blocked. For example, I should respect the elderly person's wish to stay in their own home, despite the great difficulties for health and social services in doing so, because this is where he will be able to live the life he wants to live. In this way, respect for autonomy (allowing the person to stay in his own home) contributes towards the foundations for achievement (in this case, living the desired life of independence). Equally, if I try to restrict the elderly person's choice, to coerce him into residential care, no matter how well meaning such coercion is I will be working against his health, because he will not be able to live the life he desires.

But health work, according to the values flowing from thinking of health as the 'foundations for achievement' should not be limited simply to allowing people the right of self-determination. We have a responsibility also to help *create* conditions in which individuals can actually make autonomous choices – or at least find it easier to do so. In the example above, health workers would not simply leave it up to the elderly person to decide whether he stayed in his own home or not. They would actively try to support the decision-making process, and once a course of action had been decided on, they would try to help in carrying it out. In this way, autonomy would not only be respected; it would also be created. In fulfilling these two values (autonomy respect and creation), the foundations of achievement – health – would be built.

Thinking Point

Consider Seedhouse's single value account of health – as the 'foundations for achievement'. Reflect on an example from your practice. What would you need to do in order to help create health (the 'foundations') in this particular case? How feasible is it do this? What would prevent you from doing it?

The difficulty that I identified with the 'multiple values' account of health from Downie *et al.*, is that we might well disagree about the values presented. If, however, we accept a single value account such as

Seedhouse's, we cannot then reject any of the contingent values. If I believe that health is the 'foundations for achievement', then I must also believe in the values of respecting and creating autonomy. In this sense, a Seedhouse-like argument is more coherent and unifying than a 'multiple values' account such as that of Downie and colleagues. The question now is whether we should accept the single value of health proposed. Should 'health' in fact be seen as the 'foundations for achievement'?

There are two objections to the idea that we should see it in this way:

▸ Why health as 'the foundations for achievement' rather than an alternative conception?
▸ The idea of 'foundations' might not be helpful to our practice.

The first objection is quite easy to deal with. While we can obviously conceive of health in alternative ways ('the absence of disease', say, or 'a state of complete physical, emotional and social well-being' (World Health Organisation, 1946)), this doesn't necessarily damage Seedhouse's argument. The idea of health as the 'foundations for achievement' is broad enough to include these other sorts of conceptions. For example, how can we not include the absence of disease within the 'foundations' idea? Surely adequate foundations would *include* disease absence?

The second objection is much more problematic. Its seeds are contained in the Thinking Point above. If we are potentially driven by the idea of health as the 'foundations for achievement' in our practice, how easy will it actually be to enact this value, and the further values it implies? My argument now is that the gap between a 'foundations' theory of health on the one hand, and the professional and practice culture in which it is likely to be applied on the other, is extremely wide. Given this, the theory will be both contentious and very difficult to play out in practical terms.

Much of the first part of this book was preoccupied with the critical importance of professional values and ideologies in shaping our conceptions of and responses to 'the difficulty of health studies'. What we believe, our ideologies and values, are closely enmeshed with our professional behaviours and actions. My claim is that a 'foundations' theory is so different from what might be seen as the normal run of health-related professional values and actions that putting it into practice will be enormously problematic. Most of the time, most health care professionals are responding to the requirements of services fundamentally based on the principle that their most important task is to deal with illness and disease. This is reinforced, to a great extent, by health-related public policy (Department of Health, 1997, 2000). In this sort of climate, it's reasonable to ask how possible it will be to work carefully with individuals on identifying and building on their own personal 'foundations for achievement'. The health care professional may well be more likely to go for fixing whatever the immediate problem is (the sore knee or whatever) than for assessing the extent to which 'foundations' are in place.

Think, for example, of a psychiatric nurse assessing an elderly depressed patient. The professional reaction to the patient might well be to try and manage as swiftly as possible the symptoms of the depressive illness – to regard it as a diseased state that requires quick remedy. So the nurse recommends the prescription of anti-depressant medication rather than looking more broadly to see what other possibilities might remove the obstacles and create the opportunities for achievement (cognitive behavioural therapy, say). The nurse's instinct is to deal with disease, not to contemplate 'foundations'. (This is quite apart from the economic and resource imperatives that help govern the course of action.)

The idea of professional and policy culture militating against a disposition towards 'the foundations for achievement' might apply equally as much to the areas of public health and health promotion as to acute health care. With regard to public health, the policy imperative for disease *prevention* (Department of Health, 2004), as well as professionals' own values, direct them towards particular kinds of actions. The midwife, for example, confronted with a heavily pregnant woman who smokes a pack of cigarettes a day, is probably more likely to focus on smoking as a cause of ill-health and disease than on whether the behaviour in any way contributes or not to the woman's personal 'foundations'. (It's certainly not impossible that it might do so. Smoking could be a source of comfort and support, an aid to socialisation and so on.) In these examples, and arguably in many real-life health care situations, organisational and professional imperatives overrule the possibility of attention to 'the foundations for achievement'.

Working for Health: What are we *Obliged* to Do?

Seeking agreement on the nature of values important within health care, or on the nature of health as a value itself, is a task dictated in part by our need for guidance on how we should undertake work for health. If we can agree on values or a value, then the purpose and direction of our work will be much clearer. It will be a question of working to achieve more of the value or values concerned. But our discussions have shown that getting agreement on values is a difficult task, as is acting to further them in practical settings. While this doesn't mean that we shouldn't try to do so, it does suggest that there are limits to the use of bioethics in this respect.

There is, however, an alternative bioethical approach to the form and direction of work for health that we need to consider. This is the idea that rather than attempting to achieve more of a certain value or values in our work, a more reasonable project is to propose and defend a series of *obligations* that ought to guide our activity.

The difference between this project of constructing obligations compared with that of developing accounts of health-related value or values might seem slight. Surely if we agree on the kind of value or values entailed by 'health', we are committed to certain ways of acting? This is true to an extent. However, we need to go back to the distinction I drew towards the beginning of the chapter between deontological and consequentialist theories of ethics. It's possible to imagine a situation where we are faced with a choice between creating more of the kind of *value* we associate with health (so basing our possible action on thoughts about *consequences*); or sticking to certain *obligations* (regardless of thoughts about consequences).

For example, we might believe that the nature of the value of health is the 'foundations for achievement'. Equally, we might consider that one of the obligations that ought to guide our work is a concern as far as possible to see the fair distribution of health care resources. Our actions in relation to the pregnant heavy smoker I described above may well take very different courses depending on whether we were being guided by thoughts about consequences (the maximising of the value in her individual case) or by thoughts about obligations (the concern for fair resource distribution). Maximising the value for the woman, the consequence-based approach, might suggest that we don't intervene on the question of smoking because it contributes to her 'foundations'. Concern for fair distribution of resources almost certainly demands that we would, because we know that smoking in the short term might disrupt her pregnancy, it will have an effect on the child to be born and in the end it is likely to make the mother sick. All of these things will put an unnecessary and unfair strain on health care resources. Given this, we have no option other than to strongly advise the woman against smoking.

So it's possible to see approaches to health work based on broad values and their maximisation, and approaches centred round a commitment to particular obligations as potentially being quite different. How, then, have bioethicists tried to construct such obligations? One of the most influential attempts has been the so-called Famous Four principles of health care ethics (Gillon, 1990, 1994). Within this, the obligations that become important for health care workers are:

▸ Respect for autonomy;
▸ Beneficence (the production of benefit);
▸ Non-maleficence (the avoidance of harm);
▸ Concern for justice.

Thinking Point

Those working for health should:

▸ Respect the autonomy of their patients or clients (as far as that autonomy is compatible with their own rights as autonomous beings);
▸ Attempt to produce benefit through their actions;
▸ Avoid harm;
▸ Have concern for justice in health care (e.g., through advocating or ensuring the fair distribution of scarce resources).

These principles are binding, unless one conflicts with another, in which case a choice must be made between them.

To what extent do these four principles align with your own views about what obligations exist for you as someone working for health?

What problems can you see in trying to commit to these principles?

One reason for the apparent widespread agreement with these principles is that in general they resonate with the ethical sympathies of health care workers. Broadly speaking, those working for health tend to believe that, everything else being equal, they should respect autonomy, try to produce benefit and avoid harm and be concerned about the fairness of their own actions and those of their colleagues. As Gillon, a leading exponent of the principles says:

> I have not found anyone who seriously argues that he or she cannot accept any of these. … principles or found plausible examples of concerns about health care ethics that require additional moral principles. (Gillon, 1994: 188)

There is a need to remember at this point that the task bioethics has set itself is to offer a guide as to how we should undertake work for health, both in general terms and with regard to specific activity. But there are reasons to doubt the use of the four principles approach at both of these levels:

▸ At the general level, why should there be **universal** agreement with the principles?
▸ At the specific level, individual cases may provoke a clash between principles, making it hard for the health care worker to decide what to do.

I'll consider each of these problems in turn.

The Four Principles: Is Universal Agreement Possible?

Despite the confident statements of a supporter like Gillon, although the principles might be widely accepted there is no reason why at the general level there should be universal agreement with them. Returning to the roots of ethical theory, it's possible to see the principles as stemming, once again, from a Western liberal tradition of ethics in which the autonomy of the individual takes an important place in thought and action (Duncan, 2002). But we need to note once more that this kind of tradition is not of primary importance to all societies and cultures. Some may be guided instead by traditions centred on notions of community, or of paternalism. These would give rise in turn to different sorts of principles and obligations. For example, included in the principles of a paternalistic tradition might be things like respect for wisdom and a requirement for obedience. These are obviously very different kinds of principles to those advocated by Gillon and other supporters of the 'Famous Four'.

The Four Principles: Conflict in Cases

At the level of specific activity and individual cases, it is perhaps possible to imagine all parties involved sharing a commitment to the four principles. But the problem now is of a different sort. The principles, as I've said, are binding unless one conflicts with another-in which case a choice must be made between them. Yet in all but the simplest kinds of health care activity and intervention, there is in fact likely to be conflict between principles – between, for example, respecting autonomy and producing benefit. Should we respect the pregnant smoker's autonomy and not raise the issue of smoking, or should we aim to produce the health (prevention of disease) benefit that will certainly accrue if she gives up smoking as a result of our strong advice? Conflict will occur, too, between other principles – say, between concern for justice and avoiding harm. An alcoholic seeks medical help for his sclerotic liver. If he is neglected, harm will result. (He will die.) If help is offered, the principle of justice, at least in terms of fair distribution of resources, will be offended. (Why should someone who has engaged in deliberate self-abuse get access to scarce medical treatment?)

Thinking Point

Reflect on an example from your own practice or experience. In the light of the four principles, consider which of these would have been relevant in trying to decide how to act. Would there have been conflict between principles? If you believe there would have been, analyse the cause of the conflict.

This is not to deny the importance of the ethical debate that the four principles might provoke. If, however, we are seeking definitive guides to action (as practitioners might reasonably expect), then they may well not offer us the particular help that we require (Duncan and Cribb, 1996).

Values, Health and Society

The aim of this chapter was in part to examine whether the 'sub-discipline' of ethics was able to provide us with definitive help in clarifying the nature of the value of health, or values associated with health. If clarification were possible, then we would not only be more certain about the nature of health itself, but also about the purpose of work for health. Connected to this aim, although distinctive in its own right, was the further one of trying to establish whether ethics could offer us general or particular guidance in our health work.

The response in relation to both aims has been ambiguous. We can certainly use ethical theory to flesh out the nature of health-related values and obligations. The illumination it offers might well support processes of critical analysis and reflection related to 'the difficulty of health studies'. It is, however, partial. Values will be disputed at individual, organisational and societal levels. Dispute and disagreement at different levels will make it hard to act on alternative conceptions of values.

It could be argued that dispute is inevitable because normative ethical theory and moral debate takes place in a social context. At various points in this chapter, I've deliberately emphasised the profound relationship between ethics and society; between ethical theory and the social times in which it was developed; and between normative beliefs and the cultures in which they are prominent. This has partly been to counter an assumption, often unspoken, that ethics emerges as a result of the wisdom of philosophers in ivory towers, disconnected from society (Russell, 1979).

At least part of the reason why at first glance ethics has the appearance of coming from an ivory tower is that its arguments are *a priori*. While they are constructed in a social and cultural context, they claim to convey truths that exist prior to experience of these contexts. Although *a priori* argument is often stimulating and provocative, offering challenges to and consolations for our views, it will not necessarily match with the empirical world. Maybe critical perspectives on health can be advanced through focused and careful thinking about our social world, perhaps in part through reference to empirical evidence. There is a need to think about how we as social actors, operating in (possibly operated on *by*) social structures, construct 'health', as well as why we do so. This is the purpose of the next chapter.

Turning Point?

Both kinds of projects of bioethics that I've reviewed in this chapter – attempts to establish the value of health (or values associated with it) and efforts to define the obligations of those working for health – seem to adopt a particular perspective. They both

Turning Point? *continued*

appear to suggest health-related values or obligations can be constructed and somehow 'transmitted' to health care professionals. We need to accept the values or obligations that are being in some way handed down to us. This idea is especially resonant when thinking about codes of conduct, which frequently guide health professional action and which are presented by professions as declarations of the shared values and obligations of their members. Dawson (1994) talks about codes as representative of what he calls *'outside in'* ethical thinking. Ethics is on the outside, imposed on professionals who necessarily have to accept its demands.

But this is a relatively narrow understanding of ethics. Surely as well as being subject to it as some kind of external demand, we also have the capacity to develop our own ethical sensibilities? This is what Dawson begins to talk about as *'inside out'* thinking. Presented with a particular situation, we use our developed capacity as 'moral individuals' to think about, understand and deal with the circumstances.

'Inside out' ethical thinking, developing and using the moral capacity we have within us aligns with a further theory of ethics that I have not so far discussed. This is *virtue theory*, often associated with the ancient Greek philosopher, Aristotle (384–322 BC). Aristotle's work, notably his 'Ethics' (Aristotle, 1955) is arguably different from the other theories so far examined. His claims about man's moral nature and imperatives were based on observation of the world, with the intention of assessing what it might mean to be 'virtuous'. In this sense, Aristotle was an empiricist.

For Aristotle, virtue is the mean between two extremes. Courage, for example, would neither be excessive bravery in adverse situations (this would be foolhardiness) nor undue caution (this would be cowardice). The courageous person is the one who shows the right degree of bravery, fortitude and so on in relation to the given situation. They learn what this 'right degree' is through continuous processes of reflection and contemplation on their experiences and observations.

There are many questions and difficulties associated with virtue theory. However, the theory is worth considering in the context of our discussion because it may form a way of understanding the value of health; and the obligations that we have in working for health.

Turning Point? *continued*

A virtue theory – like view of the value of health might see it as a mean between extremes. It is, for example, the possession of the right degree of autonomy, of concern for others and self, of commitment to work and leisure, of awareness of vulnerability and so on. Equally, the idea of the mean might be relevant to considering the nature of the obligations presented to health care workers. There is a need on the part of those working for health, for example, to respect autonomy to the correct extent, to observe the principles of justice insofar as they contribute in the right degree towards social equality and so forth.

The questions posed in this Turning Point are these:

▸ Does virtue theory suggest a more promising way of understanding the value or values of health?
▸ What problems are there with the idea of the mean applied to health-related values and obligations?
▸ What problems are there with the idea that moral capacity can be developed 'from within', through reflection and contemplation?

What's gone on in this chapter?

I have discussed the purpose of ethics and the use of its discourses to those who are studying health. I've argued that the distinctive ethical projects of establishing the nature of the value of health and of determining what obligations health care workers ought to have are interesting and useful – but both have limits. There seems to be a particular gap between ethics as *a priori* enquiry and the natural concerns those working for health have for guidance on dealing with the real world and its practical problems. I've ended the chapter by suggesting that a changed focus – on discourses that attempt to understand how our social world operates and how we construct it – might help move us forward in understanding 'the difficulty of health studies'.

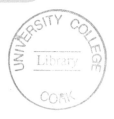

9 The Production of Health: Critical Perspectives from Sociology

What is this chapter going to do?

I move now from considering the contribution of the *a priori* discipline of philosophy (and its sub-discipline of ethics) in understanding 'the difficulty of health studies', into the domain of sociology. This latter discipline is apparently much more concerned with developing its understanding of the world through the use of empirical evidence. It aims to gather data and to analyse this so that we build responses to questions including (importantly for health studies students) questions about the production of health. How and why do social structures affect health? How and why do societies produce more (or less) health? Central to these questions is the nature of the relationship between individuals and social structures. An important idea within the sociology of health care – the idea of the all-powerful 'clinical gaze' controlling our lives and health – is discussed and critiqued. While it's possible to have some sympathy with the idea of the 'clinical gaze', arguments in its favour also present problems. We might consider that they veer too far towards an 'anti-medicine' stance within the sociology of health care, which itself is the product of sociology's ambiguous relationship with biomedicine.

Social Structures, Social Action and Health

The starting point for my discussion about ethical perspectives on health in the previous chapter was the idea that a way of understanding health is through its association with 'proper human functioning'. This had emerged in turn from the profound difficulties faced by objectivist accounts, and the only marginally less severe problems encountered by 'health is anything and everything' views of the concept. Questions in the previous chapter centred round the values that we need to promote and the obligations we must keep if we are to maintain or improve proper human functioning (and so health), addressed through the *a priori* thinking of ethics. The responses to these questions were normative; that is to say, they were attempting to establish a standard (in the form of a value or an obligation) that we should be bound to follow.

Our questions now become rather different. Instead of asking about what we *should* value and what we *ought* to do, we are interested in discovering how and why our values (and related behaviour and action) are *actually represented* in our social world. This is in part the territory of sociology, the systematic study of human society and social life (Daykin, 2001: Jones, 1994).

There is a reason for drawing the distinction between ethics and sociology rather sharply. In the context of my project of separate disciplinary explorations in search of understandings to 'the difficulty of health studies', it is to emphasise the difference of questions to be asked. It is also partly to emphasise the traditional disciplinary dichotomy between philosophy (including ethics) on the one hand and sociology on the other (and indeed the divisions between these disciplines and others). These divisions, I argued in Chapter 3, formed part of the reason for the problems faced by health studies students.

But while it's necessary to bear disciplinary division and difficulty in mind, it's also important to be reminded of the shifting context in which we are studying health and consequent changes in the orientation of disciplines. We also need to be made aware again of the plausible argument (Naidoo and Wills, 2001) for health studies to be regarded as an interdisciplinary 'field'. So increasingly within this field of health studies, it's possible to see, for example, sociologists becoming interested in philosophy (Morris, 1998) and philosophers interested in sociology (Cribb, 2005).

Nevertheless, for the reasons I've given, I need to mark out the questions that I think sociology could offer help with as we try to gain critical perspective on health:

- ▸ How and why do social structures and social action affect 'proper human functioning' (and so health)?
- ▸ How and why is more or less health produced both in and by society?

191

Central to both of these questions is a particular sociological theme I want to spend time exploring. This is the issue of the exercise of *power and control* over health. So we come up with three further questions related particularly to this theme:

▸ To what extents can individuals, groups and communities be said to have control over their own health?
▸ If control doesn't lie with those whose health it is, where does it rest?
▸ How and why has power and control been gained by others?

Thinking Point

Why might it be important to try and understand where power and control over health is located in society, and why it is located in that position?

The issue of power and control over health is fundamentally to do with the *production* of health. Depending on where control over health is located, more or less of it will be produced for individuals and communities. We can argue, too, that location of power over health is essentially related to the question of *inequalities* in health. This is one of the areas of key debate in the application of sociology to health and health care. We can argue that the presence of power and control in particular locations is more or less likely to foster or perpetuate inequalities. These arguments about power, inequalities and the production of health generally (at least to some extent) draw on actual empirical evidence gathered from particular social contexts. In this way at least, as I have said, they differ from the *a priori* claims of philosophy and ethics.

Does this pose a problem? This chapter seems to represent a sudden leap. From the contested *a priori* arguments of ethics and philosophy, I have moved to a world in which health has become a tangible, undisputed entity. After all, if I'm prepared to talk about the 'production' of health, I must surely have something in mind that counts as the 'finished product'. So it seems reasonable to ask the question, if sociologists (or at least some sociologists) are able to quantify health in some way, why are philosophers unable to do the same? At least part of this chapter's argument, though, is that sociologists might be equally susceptible as philosophers to making claims that are based more on ideologies and values than on empirical evidence. This should have the result of making us much more sceptical of sociologists who claim that they have particular insights into the nature of health and its production. If views on the location of power and control over health can (as I will argue) be disputed, so can the nature of the 'health' being fought over.

The Nature of Sociology

From before, if it's asserted that sociology is about the systematic study of human society and social life, what methodologies does it use? Broadly speaking, the methodologies of sociology revolve around:

> ▸ The collection and critical analysis of data, and;
> ▸ The testing of theory (Daykin, 2001).

These in turn give rise to a range of potential methods that sociologists might use in their work; the collection of statistical information (epidemiological or demographic details, say); survey work; question-naires; observations studies; interviews, and so on. Methodologies related to data collection and analysis on the one hand, and theory testing on the other, are of course frequently connected. We collect and analyse data at least sometimes in order to test or refine a developing theory. Equally, we develop theory in part through the analysis of data that has been gathered, and reflection on it.

Consider an example demonstrating this. Say that I'm broadly interested in the relationship between text messaging (as a 'new' form of communication) and young peoples' health. Perhaps I think that in some way text messaging might be used as a way of promoting health, or that the ability to text affects health behaviour. To begin with, I might have no firmer notion than this general interest. I begin to gather and analyse data related to the area (such as how many text messaging services have a health-related focus, how many young people use them and so on). This *data collection and analysis* might eventually lead to *theory formation* – say, my emerging theory that young people who text hold a 'health advantage' over those who don't. I may well want to test this theory through further, more specific, data collection and analysis based, for example, on comparison of the health experience and health behaviour of text messaging young people with those who don't text. Of course, there would be a need to explore the young peoples' lives quite widely in doing so, as it may well be the case that it's not text messaging as such that confers 'health advantage'. Rather it might be given by, say the greater financial resources that those young people who own mobile phones and are able to text freely have available to them.

This relatively simple example demonstrates the potential complexity of the interrelationship between data collection and analysis on the one hand, and theory testing on the other, in sociological thought and practice. It also exposes slightly further the apparent divide between modes of disciplinary approach in philosophy (including ethics) and sociology. The philosopher probably wouldn't be involved at all in this kind of complex and evolving relationship between theory and empirical evidence. Her concern instead would be to understand concepts and ideas in ways that perhaps drew from experience, but certainly didn't depend on it. This is the essential *a priori* form of philosophical thinking (Lacey, 1976). So in the text messaging and health example above, the philosopher would be trying to form and piece together what she would claim to be general truths about, say, communication and age and health, without necessarily any reference to what might be called 'reality'.

Thinking Point

Consider this particular contrast between philosophical and sociological thinking. What strengths do the interrelated methodological orientations of sociology (data analysis and theory testing) have over the *a priori* nature of philosophy? Are there weaknesses as well as strengths in these orientations with regard to exploration of 'the difficulty of health studies'?

One possible weakness of sociology's orientations lies in their potential to lead us towards believing that our careful theorising and analysis of the social world will expose a unified and authentic social 'reality'. We've consistently faced problems from the very beginning of this book with objectivist accounts of health, and constructions of our understanding based on positivist enquiry. We recognise the weaknesses in these positions and methodologies, at least as far as the elusive idea of 'health' is concerned. But there is the distinct chance that the data collection/analysis and theory testing orientations of sociology will convince us that these particular disciplinary grounds will at last help us to get to the bottom of things. The philosopher and the ethicist, someone might argue, construct *their own reality*. The sociologist, on the other hand, *engages with reality* to understand it better and to present that understanding.

The notion of a discoverable authentic reality lies at the heart of positivist conceptions of social science, and fuels the positivist *versus* anti-positivist debate within the discipline of sociology. From the bare bones of its methodological orientations towards analysis of collected data and theory testing (and the intertwining of these), it is possible for someone to move in one of two ways:

▸ They can adopt the position of the *positivist* and hold an enduring belief in the certainty of empirical observation leading us to objective facts about the world (Lacey, 1976; Jones, 1994);

▸ Or they can take an *anti-positivist* stance, emphasising the essential importance of social interaction in creating meaning in social life. Thus there are no objective truths in social understanding, only different interpretations of social action (Jones, 1994).

The separate positions of the positivist and the anti-positivist lead to particular tensions that have important implications for the application of sociology to the areas of our own interest – health and health care – which I will discuss in the following pages. They also pervade the nature and outcomes of sociological theorising. Sociologists have been centrally concerned, through their methodologies, to try and develop two different kinds of theories of social explanation:

▸ They have been concerned to develop theories related to *social structure;* how is society structured? Why is it structured in this way?

▸ They have also tried to develop theories of *social action;* how do people act? Why do they act so?

Clearly there would seem to be some kind of relationship between social structuring and individual action. A central problematic for sociology lies in trying to determine what the nature of that relationship actually is. There are at least three potential kinds of responses to this problematic:

▸ Social structures are seen as bearing (either oppressively or positively) on individuals and their actions;

▸ Individual actions are viewed as shaping and determining social structures;

▸ The relationship between individuals and their society is a dynamic one, with each interacting on the other and each having the capacity to influence and change one another (Thorogood, 2002).

Theories of Social Structure

Theories of social structure offer their accounts in terms of either *consensus* or *conflict* (Daykin, 2001). *Consensus* accounts of social structure related to health, health care and medicine importantly include the functionalist theories of Talcott Parsons (1902–1979), whose work dominated medical sociology until the 1960s. Broadly speaking, Parsons saw society as a system of interdependent parts, within which medicine was crucial in supporting and maintaining social functioning, keeping people healthy or restoring them to health so that they could continue their contribution to such functioning (Jones, 1994). For Parsons, medicine is a mechanism of control, but this control is seen positively because the social system is essentially benign.

In contrast to this, *conflict* accounts of social structure argue for our seeing society as composed of competing groups with highly vested interests, which attempt to further those interests at the expense of others. For conflict theorists, functionalism is a myth; society 'functions' for the benefit of privileged groups within it. So medicine attempts to control or subjugate other professions (such as nursing) to ensure its power and prestige (Friedson, 1970). Or conflict may be perceived as wider and much more pervasive through, say, Marxist structural theories, within which medicine is seen as a contributor to capitalist interests and an immensely strong hand in controlling health and illness, and access to health care, for the benefit of capitalism (Jones, 1994).

Theories of Social Action

Theories of social action revolve around the requirement felt by some sociologists to understand the actions and reactions of individuals and groups to society – to 'interpret the complex inter-relationships between social structures and human actions' (Jones, 1994: 47). In general terms, such theories resist the need that might be felt by social structuralists to attempt to offer decisive and all-embracing theories of social organisation. Their projects of interpretation tend to try and understand 'micro' – social situations; they involve themselves heavily in qualitative explorations and as such represent the anti-positivist tradition in sociology. *Interactionist* theories, such as those of Howard Becker and colleagues (see, for example, Becker *et al.*, 1977) view the individual as a social actor who mediates the social world. Through such mediation the conditions for shared social life and relations are created. According to interactionist theory, then, individual capacity for social action will play a central role in our accumulation of health and our resistance to ill-health. Bury (1997), for example, connects the experience of old age and the likelihood of 'being less well' with the acquisition (or perceived acquisition) of an altered social role.

Theories of the Dynamic Interaction between Individuals and Society

In beginning and focusing their explanations at the level of either structure or individual action, both social structure and social action theorists tend to be concerned with (and arguably led by) the 'macro' and 'micro' contexts that interest them. For the social structuralist, what is of interest is the 'macro' social context; for action theorists, the interest lies in individual behaviour. One result of this is a difficulty in accounting fully for the nature of the relationship between society and the individuals who inhabit it. The lens of the separate theorists is on one or the other, rather than on both.

In terms of the themes of this chapter – power and the production of health – one effect of this is that the two separate theoretical camps locate power over health in the particular context they are concerned with. The structuralist sees certain interests in society as exercising power to produce more or less health, for either benevolent or oppressive purposes. The social action theorist sees meaning (and so power) created and exercised by individuals.

But locating power in this way suggests that it is somehow a fixed commodity, which either we possess or not. Some social theorists, on the other hand, have argued that relationships (including relationships of power) between structures and individuals, as well as between different social groupings, are in fact much more fluid than this. Power should be seen as a medium for the expression of relationships rather than as a fixed commodity (Thorogood, 2002). The idea of the *social construction* of knowledge and power (this is to say that these things emerge from, and change through, the experiences and circumstances of individuals and groups) gives rise to notions of much more dynamic and shifting relationships between people and structures. So 'health' moves from being something that is structurally embedded, or part of a role (in other words, fixed) to a construction that can be disputed, altered and resisted (Foucault, 1973).

These three separate kinds of sociological theorising on the nature of social life and social meaning have important implications for the debates related to the production of health that I'll shortly consider. But before I move to these, I want to think about a general problematic connected to the use of sociology in understanding health and health care.

The Problematic in Applying Sociology in the Context of Health and Health Care

Linda Jones argues that 'it is the positivist tradition that has been the most influential in the development of sociology, and in science and medicine as well' (Jones, 1994: 45).

Thinking Point

Reflect on this statement. Considering both what Jones says and my own discussion on the nature of sociological enquiry, what could be the problematic in applying sociological thinking to an investigation of 'the difficulty of health studies'?

My discussion earlier pointed to the possibility that sociology's twin orientations towards theorising and data collection/analysis in the 'real world' will somehow lead us to believe that its methodologies will expose a unified and authentic social 'reality'. This worry might well have been dispelled in considering the range of ways in which social structures and social action have been theorised. Much of this theoretical work has emerged from, or been connected to, careful empirical analysis. There is a risk, however, that the influence of the positivist tradition on the development of sociology combined with its living in ' the shadow of biomedicine', as I have called it, with all its positivist associations, will yield relatively uncritical accounts of health and health care.

Alternatively, reactions against the positivist tradition might produce highly critically charged accounts. In other words, given history and association, the problematic lies in the balance of sociology's response to the 'difficulty of health studies'. We might adopt the long-standing position of the positivist, or we might swing completely against this, in reaction or rebellion. Is there a balance? If there is, what is it?

Until relatively recently, sociology's preoccupation with medicine, health and health care has been to provide support and justification for practices in these areas (Bunton, Nettleton and Burrows, 1995). Moreover, the power of 'the shadow of biomedicine' has led to positions where determining the objective reality of social life is pursued as a reasonable academic and policy objective. We can perhaps call this in shorthand sociology *for* health and health care. We might be able to call the opposing and much more recent tradition of critiquing health and health care-related practices, inspired partly by the development of theories of social constructionism, sociology *of* health and health care. But the division is perhaps not as neat and simple as this.

The Australian academic Deborah Lupton seems to express the internal conflict that exists within sociology applied to health, both the 'for' and the 'of' kinds. She writes, 'It is now rarely asserted within sociology that a bodily process. … is purely a product of biology' (Lupton, 1996: 1). But this shift away from narrow positivism is being undertaken in a highly difficult climate:

> While public health research is often described as 'multi-disciplinary', quantitative sociology, biostatistics, epidemiology, social psychology, demography and the stimulus-response model of communication have traditionally dominated. (Lupton, 1995: 1)

Moreover, as Lupton notes, there is a recognisable tendency for sociologists to submit the practices of mainstream medicine (and its supposed objectivity) to radical critique, while sparing more supposedly humanistic and interpretive endeavours such as health promotion from too vehement attack. It's now possible to express the problematic of applying sociology to health care more fully:

> *Can sociology, with its positivist traditions and more recent reactions against these, provide an adequate and balanced account of the nature, value and limitations of a wide range of medicine and health care-related*

policies and practices? To what extent will values and ideologies intervene?

As I've tried to make clear through this book, these kinds of questions relate not just to sociology but to other disciplines involved in the analysis of health and health care. However, they do seem particularly relevant to sociology, given the nature of the discipline's development, associations and aspirations.

Health: Power and Control

Acknowledging and understanding discourses related to the location of power and control over health is essential if we are to move forward in understanding the nature of health and how we engage in maintaining, restoring and creating it. Where does power over the production of health lie?

One possible starting point might be *us* – or rather, our bodies. Beginning at least with the ancient Greeks, the idea of the body as being healthy if it was in some way 'balanced' and regulated through lifestyle has been an important one (Williams, 2003). Responsibility for health lay with the individual, it was believed, both to maintain the balance of body, mind and spirit; and to engage in 'self-reporting' of imbalances, which played a central role in processes aimed at the restoration of health (Williams, 2003: 11). Thus the unified body (corporeal, mental and spiritual) was the source of power and control over the production or diminution of health.

The emergence of biomedicine, however, irretrievably altered this kind of conception of the source of power over health. As the corporeal body at least (in contrast with the mind, some would argue) was mapped, analysed and understood to a greater and greater extent, so the locus of power and control over health seeped *from* bodies *to* biomedical practitioners.

Increases in knowledge and understanding of the body, its mechanisms and processes grew exponentially from the time of the Enlightenment of the eighteenth century. And although medicine's capacity actually to *produce* health (that is to say, on its terms to counter and treat disease) was much less than its ability to understand the processes of the body, there nevertheless grew up a highly influential discourse promoted by biomedicine. This is the 'medical model' of health, in which as we've already discussed, health is a biological fact, reducible to the idea of parts in the 'machine' of the body going wrong and needing to be fixed by medical experts (Gillespie and Gerhardt, 1995). If we accept this discourse, then clearly power to produce health lies exclusively with those experts.

Thinking Point

The idea of the pervasiveness of the medical model of health has extended through much of this book. Now it has been located in these discussions on power and the production of health. Reflect again on your own professional role in health care. To what extent do you believe that as an 'expert' professional you have power and control over the production of health, and why?

Responses to this Thinking Point might have been mixed. On the one hand, you might have recognised the position of advantage that you hold in relation to patients or clients seeking the help you're able to offer. On the other hand, you may also have been reminded of the limits not only to your own power in the production of health but also to those of colleagues (including supposedly more influential colleagues) – and indeed the wider health care system. Given this, there is a need to reflect further on both the importance and the ambiguity of what David Armstrong has referred to as 'the clinical gaze'.

The Importance of the 'Clinical Gaze'

Armstrong (himself a clinician as well as a sociologist) offers an important analysis of the power of biomedicine as a producer of health. In his paper, 'From Clinical Gaze to Regime of Total Health' (Armstrong, 1993), he describes the emergence of biomedicine and the submission of the body to its power. Indeed, for Armstrong, the 'clinical gaze' of biomedicine actually occupies bodily spaces:

> The clinical gaze, encompassing all the techniques, languages and assumptions of modern medicine, establishes by its authority and penetration an observable and analysable space in which is crystallised that apparently solid figure of the discrete human body. (Armstrong, 1993: 56)

Drawing from Foucault, he claims that medical knowledge has in effect constructed the body. Because of this, medicine possesses sole power to deal with the body's ills. He then moves to a further, even more extensive position. Not only has the gaze of medicine constructed the body; in the twentieth-century it has also begun to move into what he calls the 'undifferentiated space between bodies' (Armstrong, 1993: 57). Health and illness, through the endeavours of activities such as epidemiology, public health and health promotion, have been constructed by medicine as entities and concerns that extend beyond bodies into *the social spaces between bodies*. Once more, as it did with the body, medicine has appropriated these spaces and claimed that it alone has the expertise to deal with illness and produce health. It has extended its gaze from the body to a 'regime of total health'. Medicine created:

> An organisational structure which could both survey and constantly monitor the whole community. (Armstrong, 1993: 58)

District nurses and health visitors, health promotion specialists and social workers, along with a range of other occupations: clinics and check-ups, screening and lifestyle records, together with a variety of other mechanisms form this regime and maintain surveillance of, and control over, our health. The 'clinical gaze', thus extended, is complete.

Armstrong's analysis is important in its demonstration of medicine's powerful involvement (and arguably dominance) in the social construction of health and illness. There is a crucial need to reflect on the apparent power of medicine to control health, and to produce more or less of it according to its own desires. Moreover, if his analysis is right, the extension of the gaze has been carefully accomplished. In terms of power, the central requirement for control over health, this has been apparently spread across a much larger and diverse range of people and occupations than was the case in the establishment of the original, body-focused medical gaze of the Enlightenment and later. The wide network of power holders (the kinds of people I referred to before) make it much less likely that medicine will be accused of monopolising power over health, although a great deal in Armstrong's argument suggests that he believes monopolisation is exactly what medicine has accomplished.

Thinking Point

What kinds of arguments would you construct both *for* and *against* Armstrong's idea of the all-encompassing 'gaze' of medicine?

The Ambiguity of the 'Clinical Gaze'

Armstrong's argument is a substantial contribution to the sociology *of* health and health care. But there is a real risk that it runs up against the problematic in applying sociology to health care that I described above – the difficulty of trying to achieve balance in understanding, given the charged atmosphere of sociology and health care. His radical critique may have ignored some aspects of the development of society and medicine that suggest the idea of the 'clinical gaze' is rather more ambiguous and difficult to isolate.

In the first place, much seems to turn in his argument on the history and chronology of medicine's development. For him, the late eighteenth century witnessed the birth of modern medicine with its capacity to map and to analyse, and so to control, the body. The nineteenth century saw the development of this power and control, such that by what seems to be the start of the twentieth century, medicine began to undertake the project of extending its 'gaze' beyond bodies to the social spaces between people. The problem with this account, though, is that it doesn't seem to take strong enough notice of earlier, pre-twentieth century versions and projects of public health. In particular, there is a need to establish the place of the great nineteenth century public health reforms within the account, and how they might affect Armstrong's conceptualisations. Should they be regarded as 'medical' reforms, in which case why do they not form part of the 'gaze'? And if they are not, what are they?

These reforms addressed the great environmental ills of Victorian Britain; providing for new means of sanitation, developing and protecting safe supplies of water and so on. To be fair to Armstrong, he does mention the nineteenth century system of public health within his argument, suggesting that at this stage 'the environment was the potential source of ill health' (Armstrong, 1993: 58). But for him, a short historical time later the focus had shifted from concerns about the environment to worries about *people* as medicine began to establish and exert its extended gaze. It is not clear why he regards the focus as changed, and his argument falters unless we accept his presumption and classification – that the public health reforms were 'environmental' rather than 'medical'. The argument falters because it depends on a clear and uninterrupted association of certain historical events (the eighteenth century 'birth' of modern medicine, the early twentieth century preoccupation with bodies and personal hygiene) with his thesis of the unstoppable onslaught of medical power.

In fact, the historical picture is much more mixed than this, with the rise of medicine running alongside increased awareness and expertise on environmental risks and how to deal with them. These formed part of nineteenth century scientific development, but we would be hard pressed necessarily to call them 'medical' developments. Or rather, if we did we would be making a choice to describe them as such that was based partly in ideology. What Armstrong seems to have done is to choose to foreground and describe particular aspects of history and attribute to these his theoretical construction of the powerful 'clinical gaze'.

There is, of course, some reason in doing so. We can point fairly easily to traditions of individual, community and population surveillance that extend through the period under review. We can connect these to the development of what for much of the last century at least was actually called 'public health *medicine*' and subject to the protectionism of medical practitioners (Webster and French, 2002). However, we can also point to other activities and traditions that have been about (or have had the consequence of) producing more health. For example, McKeown (1976) identified a range of interventions (such as improved housing, sanitation and so on) undertaken in almost exactly the same period as that described by Armstrong. He did so in order to make an empirical case for social interventions having a much greater impact on the decline of tuberculosis (TB) in the United Kingdom than medical ones, and in doing so directly dichotomised medical and social practices. TB becomes an exemplar case for the relative weakness of medicine in dealing with disease (and so by implication in producing health).

We can, of course, argue with McKeown's conception of the nature of the practices he talks about as much as we can do so with Armstrong's. The point is, though, that the choice of how to describe them is *ideological*. Armstrong's social construction of medicine's 'extended gaze' supports his belief in the power of medicine to produce (or diminish) health. McKeown's considerably more structural argument implicitly locates a range of different kinds of power within structures. We can argue productively about the degrees and relative influence of power at levels of both social action and social structure, but it is necessary to acknowledge that ideologies underpin all such arguments. Perhaps we can also wonder why the idea of 'health', as this book has attempted to understand and conceptualise it, is so under-represented in these kinds of arguments.

It's possible to assert that Armstrong's argument is essentially about medicine, while McKeown's relates to disease. Why do both writers apparently find it so difficult within their analyses to talk about 'health', as the idea has been developed in the arguments of this book?

Connecting the Importance and the Ambiguity of the 'Clinical Gaze' through the Idea of the 'Health Consumer'

We have now considered both the importance of a 'clinical gaze', social constructionist account of power and health; and the difficulties inherent in this kind of theorising. It certainly seems crucial to consider medicine as an essential location of 'power over health'. However, there might also be a tendency on the part of sociologists of medicine to locate power relations too firmly in the structures of surveillance created and maintained by medical practitioners, apparently with the willing connivance of the range of health care-related occupations. After all, if power is seen in Foucauldian terms as a medium through which relations are expressed, as something that is circulating rather than fixed, then we need to pay attention to others involved in medical and health care relationships. We need especially to consider the layperson, characterised on occasions as 'the patient'.

Something important seems to have happened to this person over the last part of the twentieth century and into the twenty-first. It is that (in affluent, Western societies at least), she has become more preoccupied with her 'health'. And this preoccupation has taken the form of a concern to integrate whatever choices exist around health into lifestyle and senses of personal identity (Scambler, 2002). As Bunton, Nettleton and Burrows note:

> In the 1960s a list of 'health-related' commodities would have included items such as aspirins, TCP, Dettol and plasters. Today, however, it would include: food and drink; myriad health promoting pills; private health; alternative medicine; exercise machines and videos; health insurance; membership of sport and health clubs; walking boots; running shoes and so on. (Bunton, Nettleton and Burrows, 1995: 1–2)

One way of understanding this change in the context of the 'disorganised capitalism' that exists at the turn of the millennium is as a commercial expansion connected to an 'ideology of consumerism' (Scambler, 2002: 130). But if the layperson has become the 'health consumer', we need to ask where power now lies. Is it with this relatively new consumer? Is it with medical practitioners? Or does it lie somewhere else altogether?

For David Armstrong, the answer to these questions is clear. This new consumer of health has been recruited by medicine to 'monitor their own bodies' (Armstrong, 1993: 63). Lifestyles have been appropriated with the purpose of supporting the control of disease – the task of medicine (and this task is the source of medicine's social legitimacy and power). In our concern with health as a 'lifestyle accessory', the blurring of health and disease becomes increasingly common. In health, we are also 'at risk' from disease, a risk that we cannot afford because 'health' (the alternative medicine, health clubs and so on of Bunton *et al.*'s conceptualisation) represents so much of our identity as consumers. And in our concern to avoid 'risk' and so preserve identity, we become willing subjects for the exercise of power and control.

In a sense, this latter-day idea of the creation of the 'health consumer' brings us back to the notion with which we began this discussion of power and control over our health – our bodies. In ancient Greece, the individual largely held domain over his (unified) body. In the early twenty first century, we are encouraged (someone like Armstrong might argue that we are coerced) into possession of control over our body, because we are consumers of health. The notion of bodies consuming 'health products' and thereby producing health is one way of connecting both the importance and the ambiguity of the 'clinical gaze'.

There seems little doubt that the 'gaze' is an important feature in the establishment of ourselves as 'health consumers' (Bunton, Nettleton and Burrows, 1995). On the other hand, to suggest that the forces by which we are willingly (or otherwise) led into the roles of consumers depend solely on medicine for their generation seems too much to claim, even if we accept the profound power of medical practices and discourse. As I argued before, medicine is simply one of a number of social forces that conspire to make us frequently act as we do – that is to say, as conspicuous and consuming bodies (Glassner, 1995).

On the basis of the emerging account of health and influences on its conceptualisation that has been developed in this book, where do you think power over health is located?

▸ Is it with medical practitioners?
▸ Is it with other health care-related occupations?
▸ Is it with the lay-person as health consumer?
▸ Or is it located somewhere else entirely?

Attempt to justify to yourself your analysis and decision about the location of 'power over health'.

The Production of Health

The idea that in some way individuals and structures are involved in the production of health is an important one. There are two different aspects to this importance.

▸ First, we need to have a practical concern with the idea because in developing conceptions of how individuals understand and shape their own health (and the health of others), and the shaping influence of structures, we will help ourselves in supporting the production of 'more health'. If we believe, say, that aspects of social structure such as income, housing, education and clean air and water contribute to health, then understanding how these are controlled and how it's possible to influence control will assist in attempts to modify negative effects on health. It will also, of course, support efforts to control structures so that they contribute to 'more health'. Perhaps this is what lies behind attempts (e.g., Wilkinson, 1996) to investigate the notion of 'inequalities in health' and present it in positivist terms as an empirical reality that can (and ought to be) addressed through policy and practice.

▸ Second, if we suggest that the production of health depends on the actual location of power over health and the nature of power relationships, then it strongly implies a need to establish whether or not we are happy with this location of power. This aspect is different because it is *ideological*. Are we happy, for example, with the idea of the 'extended clinical gaze' and (from Armstrong) the shaping of ourselves within this into constantly self-monitoring and self-surveying consumers of health? There is no necessary reason why we should feel uncomfortable with this idea. After all, the payback for us might be that we maintain (or improve) levels of health (quite probably not only in terms of absence of disease but also with regard to the 'proper human functioning' argument we've been pursuing) that will be beneficial.

However, it could also be the case that we are in fact unhappy about the location of power over the production of health with which we are presented. Why should we agree, for example, with health care professionals trying to exercise such substantial control over our health, apparently without negotiation? Why should we accept that relative degrees of power over health bestowed by virtue of the class or ethnic or gender position that we occupy (and thus our susceptibility or otherwise to health inequality) be allowed to continue?

We are in a position either to agree or to disagree with the nature of the relationship between individuals, social structures and health. And in assuming the position that we do, we are adopting a set of values. For example, if I agree that inequalities in health are a result of natural selection (because of someone's genetic makeup, say, they are more susceptible to shorter, more unhealthy lives), I am committing myself to a certain view of the world. This is a view in which some are placed at inevitable and unavoidable natural disadvantage. In an important sense, it doesn't matter whether or not genetics plays an empirical part in the creation of inequalities. What matters is that I choose to accept this and what it says about being human. (Natural selection means that not all humans are equal.) In this acceptance, I also make certain choices about the practical part I should play in the production of health. For example, I impose (or agree to the imposition of) certain limits in my work for health that take account of the idea of natural selection. In this way, the ideological and practical aspects of the importance of ideas about how health is produced are drawn together.

The fact that ideas on the production of health involve values connects this particular debate with the discussions of the previous chapter about the value of health itself and about the obligations we have in our work for health. These all in turn relate back to the issues of professional identity and disciplinary diversity that we discussed in Part I. We need to try and draw together the range of critical and reflective perspectives on health that I have tried to explore and consider how they might continue to be developed, beyond the confines of this book.

Turning Point?

This is not so much a turning point as a place at which to begin attempts at connection and consolidation.

I have discussed a number of disciplinary attempts to be clearer about the *nature* of health; about the kinds of *values* that the concept might contain, represent or be associated with; and about how health might be *constructed* and *produced*. Before you begin to read the final chapter, and my own attempts to suggest how we might develop these various perspectives on health, it would be useful to engage in development of your own ideas about moving forward with critical perspectives on health. With the benefit of your own critical analyses of the arguments that I've presented and tried to develop, and critical reflection on your own understanding or practice, consider the following:

▸ What is your understanding now of the nature of health?
▸ If health has this nature, what does it say or imply about the value or values that we need to ascribe or relate to it?
▸ What in turn does this mean for understanding of how health is controlled and produced? Can we locate power over production in particular places? Are we happy (given our ascription of health's values and our conceptions of its nature) with such location? If not, where *ought* power and the capacity to produce health be located?
▸ What capacity do we have ourselves to shift and influence sources of power and power relations?

Although I've set these questions down in a linear form, it's highly possible that responses to one question may demand that we go back and reconsider replies to others. For example, if I see health being produced (or diminished) through certain kinds of power relationships, this may force me to reassess the kinds of values that I want to associate with health. The questions form a guide, but how you use and respond to them is down to your own analytic and reflective exploration.

What's gone on in this chapter?

In this chapter I have considered the potential contribution of sociology to understanding problems inherent within the study of health. I have considered especially sociological debates around the production and control of health by medicine. Issues of power and control over health are complicated by different theoretical interpretations on the part of sociologists about the nature of the relationship between individuals and social structures. Moreover, the ambiguous relationship that has developed in recent times between sociology and medicine – from servant to (as some might see it) rebel – has created a problem for assessing the worth of sociology's contribution to addressing 'the difficulty of health studies'. Just how far does ideology rather than evidence drive an argument such as David Armstrong's for the supposedly arresting importance of medicine's 'clinical gaze'?

10 Developing Critical Perspectives on Health

What is this chapter going to do?

In this final chapter, I review the reasons for the approach I have taken to dealing with problems inspired by the study of health. I emphasise again the worth of developing critical perspectives on health for both academic study and practice. I suggest ways in which the process of understanding can continue and develop beyond the confines of this book.

Revisiting 'the Difficulty of Health Studies'

This book began with a cluster of questions, all centring round the essential and perplexing one of 'What is health?' A key task for health studies students is to come to some understandings and positions on this question so that they have a base from which to build responses to the 'questions cluster'. Unless we have thought about what health actually is, I've tried to argue, it will be much more difficult to respond to further questions such as 'What is the purpose of health care?' and 'How is it possible to create more health?' In fact, asking these questions doesn't really make sense unless we are prepared to spend time responding to the first, essential one of what it is that we're actually talking about.

The 'raw material' that we have to hand as we try to respond to these questions are:

▸ Our professional understanding and persona;
▸ The health-related academic discourses that we encounter.

Yet both of these are centrally implicated, I've argued, in the problem of getting a clear-sighted perspective on the questions. They are key suspects in what I have called 'the difficulty of health studies'. They have become suspects because of the highly pervasive ideologies and values contained within their character, their practices and their discourses. So ideologies and values frame and pervade the *content* of health studies. (Think, for example, of Armstrong's construction of power relations in medicine and health care, discussed in the previous chapter). But they also pervade the *process* of studying health. (Consider how difficult it might be, say, for someone who has undergone socialisation into a health-related profession not to allow the impact of this to influence their views on the nature of health.) As I discussed in Part I, the relationship between content and process in constructing 'the difficulty of health studies' is dense, complex and obfuscating. We need to come to terms with both supposedly rational argument and with quite possibly unexpressed but nevertheless all-encompassing values.

Answers? What Answers?

The resources I've proposed that we need to deal with the arguments of health studies are the twin 'tools' of critical analysis and critical reflection:

▸ We need critical analysis to dissect argument;
▸ We need critical reflection to understand our reactions to arguments and discussion, in terms of our own emotions, feelings and values (as well as those of others).

We have to recognise the worth of both cognition and affection in making sense of 'the difficulty of health studies'. If we are to engage in 'whole person' learning with regard to the study of health (which must be the case, given what such study means), we must develop ourselves as both critical analysts and critical reflectors. Analysis must be accompanied by reflection, and *vice versa*. For our purposes, the two are inseparable.

But as our discussions on the various disciplinary contributions to understanding the nature, the value and the production of health have shown, neither these contributions nor our related analyses and reflections will necessarily produce 'answers' to our questions. Or at least they won't produce answers in the sense of uncontested clarification on the issues that are troubling us. There will always be disagreements; other ways of thinking about what health is, about how we might express it as a value (or the values that might be associated with it) and about ways and means of exerting power and control in the production of health. Uncontested answers in our field don't exist (except *possibly* in relation to some narrow, technically specific matters).

> *Given this, the question then becomes, 'In the field of health studies, what kind of answers should we expect?'*

The answer to this question about answers lies in understanding both the nature of 'the difficulty of health studies' and the scope of the resources of critical analysis and reflection that we use to deal with it. Careful analysis and reflection will allow us as close observation as possible of the enmeshed issues of content and process that make up the difficulty. They will help us to establish why people have said, and continue to say, what they do about health, its nature and value and the means of its creation. They will support us in understanding our own reactions to these discourses and in evaluating the worth of our own developing accounts of health.

Together with a commitment to honest encounters with disciplines claiming to illuminate the field of our interest, this is all that analysis and reflection can do. For some, that might be depressing. What is the point in striving so hard to reach such limited understanding of so important a concept? My own view, and one that I hope you will share after having read this far, is that this kind of understanding is not limited at all. It actually constitutes quite a lot. To be able to understand and appraise the basis (in rational thought and argument, and in ideologies and values) of contest around the idea of 'health' seems to be important in itself. It also provides the ground for further work in clarifying our purpose and intention in working for health.

Thinking Point

Make a brief self-assessment of the worth of the critical perspectives developed in this book to your own developing understanding of the idea of health, and the nature and purpose of health-related work. Has the process of reading, thinking and reflecting been helpful or not? As well as making a judgement itself, try and *justify* this judgement.

The Importance of Dialogue

I've argued consistently throughout this book that 'the difficulty of health studies' is at its heart a difficulty essentially related to competing ideologies and values. It is compounded by these values and ideologies manifesting themselves in both the content of the field and in the processes by which we attempt to tackle its messy territory. Sometimes values are made explicit (for example in the ethical debates encountered in Chapter 9). Mostly they are held implicit at best, hidden (either deliberately or unwittingly) at worst. To return to the debate with which this book began; objectivist *versus* interpretivist conceptions of the nature of health. Now with the benefit of hindsight, it's possible to see that beneath the objectivist account of a writer such as JG Scadding lies a welter of values. He is not simply saying, 'Disease is objectively describable, therefore so is health – it is the absence of disease'. His argument is also expressing values preferences about a number of things:

▸ About how health should be maintained and improved;
▸ About who should be controlling its maintenance and production;
▸ About who should be complying with the controllers;
▸ About how policy should be conceived;
▸ And about how practice should be executed.

Equally an interpretivist, like David Seedhouse, is expressing his particular values preferences, which to some extent at least are likely to conflict with those of an objectivist such as Scadding.

We can trace these kinds of values conflicts back, as I have tried to do so in this book, to professional backgrounds, to disciplinary discourses, to separate constructions of – and reactions to – academic, occupational and social histories. So we return to the intertwining of values as content on the one hand, and as process on the other, that is constantly exhibited in the field of health studies. In itself, this intertwining is not necessarily negative. We cannot expect health, a fundamental human preoccupation, to be immune to separate sets of ideologies, values and interests. What is a problem is when values remain hidden or unexplored. It is problematic because neither the values themselves nor the different theoretical and practical positions that flow from them will be properly understood. They will appear as unyielding; those who hold and enact them will be seen as nothing more than plain obstinate.

This emphasises the need for *dialogue* as part of a strategy for examining and understanding perspectives on health. The more it's possible to talk to others, both from our own and from different occupations, the more likely it is that we will be able to recognise separate values – related positions and the motivations to which they give rise. We will be in a position to begin to understand why, for example, a colleague practitioner might be committed to a course of action that seems to be disruptive of a particular patient's or client's autonomy. In dialogue, we may be able to establish the importance for them of health as an objectively describable value and of their professional orientation towards producing more of that value. It's possible that we will be able to relate our different positions to separate theoretical accounts of health, its value and the nature of its production. We may still disagree with the values and actions of our colleague, but we will understand what is going on and this in turn will lead to an extended view of health and the conduct of health care.

In talking of the importance of dialogue, I mean to refer not only to dialogue with others, but also with ourselves. We need to develop and sustain the practice of self-examination, and constructing dialogues with ourselves is one way of accomplishing this. I wrote in Chapter 6 of the potential within both 'monological' and 'dialogical' reflection to move us towards greater understanding. My claim now is that with the help of the material generated in our examination of disciplinary perspectives on health, we should be in a position to begin framing our own 'internal dialogues' on 'the difficulty of health studies'.

To what extent, for example, can we agree with the kind of consensus account of the worth of medicine and health care offered by a functionalist such as Parsons? Ideologically, we may find ourselves closer in position to Armstrong's construction of medicine's 'regime of total health', but by testing alternatives against our preferred position, through 'dialogues' with ourselves, we strengthen that standpoint. We may choose to engage in self – 'dialogue' through, say, building up a series of written notes presenting position and counter-position. We may do it through forming a collection of annotated journal papers offering arguments that we both agree and disagree with. However it's done, the important outcome of 'dialogues with ourselves' is that we are always reminded there are alternative ways of thinking.

Thinking Point

How might it be possible for you to go about beginning to establish (or develop) dialogues with others; and 'dialogues' with yourself?

Studying Health and Staying Sane

Establishing a range of discussive dialogues may well not be easy. For a whole range of reasons, from lack of time to concerns about what might result from critical engagement, others may not want or feel able to involve themselves in discussion with you on the kinds of questions that this book has attempted to address. Equally, constantly prompting yourself into imagined alternative ways of thinking might be exhausting. Sometimes (perhaps quite often), we simply want to take the easy path. This is perfectly reasonable. We all need to preserve our own health. We all need to try and stay sane!

I would hope that if you are engaged in health studies, and if you've taken the trouble to reach what is almost the end of this book, you will want to use at least some of the opportunities presented to you for critical debate, analysis and reflection. If you're engaged in a formal programme of study (either face to face, or at a distance in some way), maybe an agreement you can reach with yourself is to use *this* as the prime opportunity to develop and hone critical perspectives. Perhaps you might also agree with yourself at the same time that engaging in debate in more 'difficult' contexts (e.g., your workplace) is a process that you will build up over a period of time, or save for the future. There is no point in exhausting yourself. Move forward as you feel you can. Don't regret the opportunities that you didn't take to question, to analyse, to adopt critical positions – especially if these missed opportunities related to difficult or even hostile contexts. We all have our reasons for not putting our head above the parapet on at least some occasions; and they are mostly good ones!

Equally though, the preservation of sanity while involved in the highly demanding area of health studies depends on a further principle. It is that doubt itself is valuable (Bonnett, 2001). It is certainly true that doubting can be exhausting, distressing and disturbing. It can cause you to confront your purpose and motives in ways that might well be uncomfortable. It can give rise to sleepless nights. That is why I have encouraged you to think about the limits that you might want to set for yourself in terms of your engagement with critical perspectives on health. But doubt is also challenging and exhilarating. Asking questions, confronting uncertainties, probing further and deeper into concepts, ideas and practices that have previously always been taken for granted can be enormously fulfilling. It is this sort of positive challenge that is another way of maintaining sanity in a perplexing world; one that I hope to some extent you will accept as you recognise the reward in tackling the difficulty of studying health.

What's gone on in this chapter?

I've reviewed the reasons for this book and the processes and issues it's explored to better understand 'the difficulty of health studies'. I've outlined the importance of two things in particular – engaging in dialogue (with yourself and with others) and knowing your limits – as you move forward in the exciting and challenging field of health studies.

Glossary: Key Words for Critical Perspectives on Health

This glossary provides a quick reference point for some of the key terms used in the main text. The terms and their meanings are explained and developed within the text itself, but the glossary is designed to enable you to check or refer to a meaning, as you need to do so.

Analogy. Drawing similarity between two apparently different things. An argument by analogy works by drawing attention to claims of similarity between two apparently dissimilar things and then using this claimed similarity to advance a position. Analogies are often used within arguments, but as Bonnett (2001: 103) notes, while interesting and suggestive, arguments rooted in analogy alone are not necessarily reliable.

Analysis. The process of breaking something down into its component parts so that it can be better understood.

A priori. Roughly, this means 'prior to experience'. An argument is *a priori* if it is constructed independent of experience. It contrasts with an argument based on empirical evidence of some kind.

Concept. To have a concept of something is to be able to think about that thing and be able to differentiate it from other things (Lacey, 1976: 34). I have a concept of 'mountain', say, because I can think of things that are mountains and differentiate them from other things (hills, plains and so on). Conceptual difficulty emerges in part because in relation to some concepts (e.g., 'health') there is nothing in the empirical world we can definitively point to as a basis for agreement or disagreement about the nature of the concept concerned.

Condition (necessary). A condition (for the existence of something, or agreement with an argument) is necessary if it has to be in place for us reasonably to agree with the thing's existence, the argument etc. For example, oxygen is a necessary condition for human life. Oxygen cannot be a *sufficient* condition for human life because other conditions are also required for life, such as water. (See the entry following on 'sufficient condition'.)

Condition (sufficient). A sufficient condition (for the existence of something, or agreement with an argument) is that given which it is sufficient for the thing to exist, the argument to be agreed with etc. For example, lack of oxygen is a sufficient condition for death to take place in humans. It is a sufficient condition because nothing else is needed for death to occur. (See the preceding entry on 'necessary condition'.)

Consequentialism. Systems of ethics (e.g., utilitarianism) arguing that concern for consequences should be the guide of our action.

Deontology. Systems of ethics that require us to believe in the rightness or goodness of certain actions or duties regardless of the consequences that might follow from the performance of that action or duty in a particular situation.

Discourse. A way of talking and/ or writing that has as its purpose attempts to make greater sense of the world. Some theorists see discourses as ways that social groups organise themselves so that life is better recognised and understood for that group (Holliday, 2002). This would provide a reasonable basis for starting to describe *academic discourse*. Marshall and Rowland (1998: 32), for example, describe discourse as the language, vocabulary and methods used by an academic discipline to develop and present its arguments.

Empirical. Based on experience. An argument or evidence is empirical if it is based on experience.

Enlightenment. The Eighteenth century movement whose proponents, as a result of advances in scientific explanation, came to believe and declare that all aspects of our existence could be explained through rational scientific method.

Epistemology. Branch of philosophy concerned with establishing and justifying what we can know and how we can know it. Often more-generally used as a term embracing any justification (whether based in philosophy or not) of the positions we take on the knowledge we have and how we've gathered it.

Ethics. Branch of philosophy concerned with enquiry into how we ought to act, and what we ought to regard as valuable.

Heuristics. A set of general procedures used by those working in an academic discipline to help them progress in uncovering knowledge and developing understanding (in the discipline's terms).

Ideology. Set of principles connecting how we see the world to explicit moral values. These perceptions and values are claimed by those holding them to be better than any alternative.

Interpretivism. Positions on the nature or existence of something (e.g., health) suggesting that our knowledge and understanding of that thing depends on how we interpret it.

Method. A particular technique for exploring and researching the world (especially the empirical world) – for example interviews, observations, surveys and so on.

Methodology. An account of method; this is very often of how attempts at empirical discovery were undertaken, but could also include how other (possibly related) processes such as writing and argument were developed.

Naturalism. A method of enquiry that operates with the belief that reality is relatively straightforward and can be captured by the researcher, given long and careful enough work.

Nominalism. The belief that a concept can be defined and understood by relating words or other symbols to things subject to empirical observation.

Normative. Theory and argumentation that is normative attempts to argue or theorise on the basis of prescribed norms or standards already assumed by the person arguing or theorising (Lacey, 1976).

Objectivism. Positions on the nature or existence of something (e.g., health) suggesting that we can know objective, indisputable facts about that thing.

Ontology. Branch of philosophy concerned with establishing the nature of something and developing/justifying particular accounts of its nature. Often more generally used as a term embracing any account or justification (whether based in philosophy or not) of something's existence.

Paradigm. While this term has a number of uses (Bonnett, 2001), it is employed in this book to describe a major argument that tries to assert we should see and understand the world (or an aspect of the world) in a particular way (e.g., the 'positivist paradigm').

Positivism. Positivist enquiry is that whose limits are set by what can be firmly established through empirical observation and scientific method (Lacey, 1976).

Progressivism. A general term used to embrace a range of paradigms of enquiry, all operating with the belief that reality is not 'out there', waiting to be discovered, but rather that the social world is constructed by those who live in it and those who research it.

Qualitative. Methods of investigation, enquiry and research that attempt to understand perceptions, emotions and feelings. These are to be contrasted with *quantitative* methods.

Quantitative. Methods of investigation, enquiry and research that involve *counting* and *measuring* – for example, surveys and experiments. Their philosophical basis lies in *positivism*.

Utlilitarianism. A consequentialist theory of ethics proposing moral action is that which leads to the greatest benefit for the greatest number.

Virtue theory. An ethical theory attributed to the Greek philosopher Aristotle, proposing that we learn to lead a virtuous (moral) life by recognising and acting according to the mean between two extremes (e.g., courage is the mean between foolhardiness and caution). It is sometimes referred to as 'Aristotelianism'.

References

Ackroyd, E (1984). A rejection of doctors as moral guides. *Journal of Medical Ethics*, **10**, 147.

Ahmad, WIU (ed.) (1993). *'Race' and Health in Contemporary Britain*. Buckingham: Open University Press.

Andrain, CF and Apter, DE (1995). *Political Protest and Social Change*. Basingstoke: Macmillan.

Aristotle (1955). *Ethics* (translated by JAK Thomson). Harmondsworth: Penguin.

Armstrong, D (1983). *Political Anatomy of the Body*. Cambridge: Cambridge University Press.

Armstrong, D (1993). From clinical gaze to regime of total health. In Beattie, A *et al.* (eds). *Health and Well-Being: A Reader*. Basinsgtoke: Macmillan/Open University, 55–67.

Armstrong, D (2003). Social theorizing about health and illness. In Albrecht, GL, R Fitzpartick and S Scrimshaw (eds). *The Handbook of Social Studies in Health and Medicine*. London: Sage, 24–35.

Baelz, P (1979). Philosophy of health education. In Sutherland, I (ed.). *Health Education: Perspectives and Choices*. London: George Allen and Unwin.

Ball, SJ (1990). Self-doubt and soft data: social and technical trajectories in ethnographic fieldwork. *Qualitative Studies in Education*, **3**, 2, 157–171.

Ball, SJ (2003). *Class Strategies and the Education Market*. London: Routledge Falmer.

Barker, J (2004). Reflection in mental health nursing. In Tate, S and M Sills (eds). *The Development of Critical Reflection in the Health Professions*. London: Higher Education Academy Health Sciences and Practice Subject Centre, 70–75.

Barr, H (2002). *Interprofessional Education: Today, Yesterday and Tomorrow*. London: Higher Education Academy Health Sciences and Practice Subject Centre.

Beauchamp, TH and Childress, JF (1994). *Principles of Biomedical Ethics* (Third Edition). New York: Oxford University Press.

Beck, U (1992). *Risk Society: Towards a New Modernity*. Newbury Park, CA: Sage.

Becker, HS, B Geer, EC Hughes and AL Strauss (1977). *Boys in White: Student Culture in Medical School*. New Brunswick, NJ: Transaction Books.

Becker, MH (ed.) (1984). *The Health Belief Model and Personal Health Behaviour*. Thorofare, NJ: Charles B Slack.

Beevor, A (1999). *Stalingrad*. London: Penguin.

Benton, T (1991). Biology and social science: why the return of the repressed should be given a (cautious) welcome. *Sociology*, 25, 1, 1–29.

Benner, P (1984). *From Novice to Expert: Excellence and Power in Clinical Nursing Practice*. Menlo Park, CA: Addison-Wesley.

Benzeval, M, K Judge and M Whitehead (eds) (1995). *Tackling Inequalities in Health: An Agenda for Action*. London: King's Fund.

Blackburn, C (1991). *Poverty and Health: Working with Families*. Milton Keynes: Open University Press.

Blaxter, M (1990). *Health and Lifestyles*. London: Routledge.

Blaxter, M and E Paterson (1982). *Mothers and Daughters: A Three Generational Study of Health, Attitudes and Behaviour*. London: Heineman Educational Books.

Bonnett, A (2001). *How to Argue*. Harlow: Pearson Education.

Boud, D, R Keogh and D Walker (1985). *Reflection: Turning Experience into Learning*. New York: Kogan Page.

Bourdieu, P (1986). *Distinction: A Social Critique of the Judgement of Taste*. London: Routledge.

Brown, PA and SM Piper (1995). Empowerment or social control? Differing interpretations of psychology in health education. *Health Education Journal*, 54, 115–123.

Bunton, R and G Macdonald (eds) (2002). *Health Promotion: Disciplines, Diversity and Developments* (Second Edition). London: Routledge.

Bunton, R, S Nettleton and R Burrows (eds) (1995). *The Sociology of Health Promotion: Critical Analyses of Consumption, Lifestyle and Risk*. London: Routledge.

Burleigh, M (2001). *The Third Reich: A New History*. London: Pan Macmillan.

Burns, S and C Bulmann (eds) (2000). *Reflective Practice in Nursing: The Growth of the Professional Practitioner* (Second Edition). Oxford: Blackwell Science.

Bury, M (1997). *Health and Illness in a Changing Society*. London: Routledge.

Calnan, M and B Johnson (1985). Health, health risks and inequalities: an exploratory study of womens' perceptions. *Sociology of Health and Illness*, 14, 2, 233–254.

Cedar, SH with J Hubbard (2001). Physiology. In Naidoo, J and J Wills (eds). *Health Studies: An Introduction*. Basingstoke: Palgrave, 9–38.

Chalmers, AF (1982). *What is this Thing Called Science?* (Second Edition). Milton Keynes: Open University Press.

Claxton, G (1988). *Live and Learn: An Introduction to the Psychology of Growth and Change in Everyday Life*. Milton Keynes: Open University Press.

Clouder, L (2003). Becoming professional: exploring the complexities of professional socialisation in health and social care. *Learning in Health and Social Care*, **2**, 4, 213–222.

Clouder, L (2004). Concluding overview: key points and future developments in reflective practice within the education of health professionals. In Tate, S and M Sills (eds). *The Development of Critical Reflection in the Health Professions*. London: Higher Education Academy Health Sciences and Practice Subject Centre, 101–108.

Cooter, R (2000). The ethical body. In Cooter, R and J Pickstone (eds). *Medicine in the Twentieth Century*. London: Harwood Academic Publishers.

Cornwell, J (1984). *Hard-Earned Lives: Accounts of Health and Illness from East London*. London: Tavistock.

Cox, BD (1987). *The Health and Lifestyle Survey: Preliminary Report*. Cambridge: The Health Promotion Research Trust.

Cox, BD (1993). *The Health and Lifestyle Survey: Seven Years On*. Cambridge: The Health Promotion Research Trust.

Creme, PR and MV Lea (1997). *Writing at University*. Buckingham: Open University Press.

Cribb, A (1986). Politics and health in the school curriculum. In Rodmell, S and A Watt (eds). *The Politics of Health Education: Raising the Issues*. London: Routledge and Kegan Paul.

Cribb, A (2005). *Health and the Good Society: Setting Healthcare Ethics in Social Context*. Oxford: Oxford University Press.

Cribb, A and S Bignold (1999). Towards the reflexive medical school: the hidden curriculum and medical education research. *Studies in Higher Education*, **24**, 2, 195–209.

Cribb, A and P Duncan (2002). *Health Promotion and Professional Ethics*. Oxford: Blackwell Science.

Dawson, AJ (1994). Professional codes of practice and ethical conduct. *Journal of Applied Philosophy*, **11**, 2, 145–153.

Daykin, N (2001). Sociology. In Naidoo, J and J Wills (eds). *Health Studies: An Introduction*. Basingstoke: Palgrave, 101–132.

Department of Health (1997). *The New NHS: Modern, Dependable*. London: The Stationery Office.

Department of Health (2000). *The NHS Plan*. London: The Stationery Office.

Department of Health (2004). *Choosing Health*. London: Department of Health.

Dewey, J (1974). *John Dewey on Education: Selected Writings* (ed. RD Archambault). Chicago, Ill: University of Chicago Press.

Dietitians' Board (of the Council of Professions Supplementary to Medicine) (2000). *Pre-Registration Education and Training Manual*. London: British Dietetic Association.

Downie, RS (1990). Ethics in health education: an introduction. In Doxiadis, S (ed.). *Ethics in Health Education*. Chichester: Wiley.

Downie, RS and J Macnaughton (2001). Images of health. In Heller, T *et al.* (eds). *Working for Health*. London: Sage/The Open University, 11–15.

Downie, RS, C Tannahill and A Tannahill (1996). *Health Promotion: Models and Values* (Second Edition). Oxford: Oxford University Press.

Duncan, P (2001). Ethics and law. In Naidoo, J and J Wills (eds). *Health Studies: An Introduction*. Basingstoke: Palgrave, 101–132.

Duncan, P (2002). Values, obligations and 'good lives': how useful is bioethics to sex educators? *Sex Education*, **2**, 2, 133–144.

Duncan, P (2005). Helping students learn. *DOPSE-TEMPUS Workshop*, University of Cairo, 7–8 May.

Duncan, P and A Cribb (1996). Helping people change: an ethical approach? *Health Education Research*, **11**, 3, 339–348.

Dworkin, R (1995). *Life's Dominion: An Argument about Abortion and Euthanasia*. London: Harper Collins.

Easton, D (1953). *The Political Process*. New York: Knopf.

Edmondson, R and C Kelleher (eds) (2000). *Health Promotion: New Discipline or Multi-Discipline?* Dublin: Irish Academic Press.

Eisner, E (1985). *The Educational Imagination: On Design and Evaluation of School Programs* (Second Edition). New York: Macmillan.

English National Board for Nursing, Midwifery and Health Visiting (1987). *Managing Change in Nurse Education-Pack One: Preparing for Change*. London: ENB.

Eraut, M (1994). *Developing Professional Knowledge and Competence*. London: Falmer.

Eraut, M (2002). Editorial. *Learning in Health and Social Care*, **1**, 1, 1–6.

Fade, S (2004). Reflection and assessment. In Tate, S and M Sills (eds). *The Development of Critical Reflection in the Health Professions*. London: Higher Education Academy Health Sciences and Practice Subject Centre, 76–81.

Fairbairn, G and C Winch (1998). *Reading, Writing and Reasoning: A Guide for Students* (Second Edition). Buckingham: Open University Press.

Foucault, M (1973). *The Birth of the Clinic*. London: Tavistock.

Francome, C and D Marks (1996). *Improving the Health of the Nation: The Failure of the Government's Health Reforms*. London: Middlesex University Press.

Freire, P (1972). *Pedagogy of the Oppressed*. London: Penguin.

Friedson, E (1970). *Profession of Medicine: A Study in the Sociology of Applied Knowledge*. New York: Dodd Mead.

Gabe, J and M Calnan (2000). Health care and consumption. In Williams, S, J Gabe and M Calnan (eds). *Health, Medicine and Society: Key Theories, Future Agendas*. London: Routledge.

Gallie, WB (1956). Essentially contested concepts. *Proceedings of the Aristotelian Society*, 1956, 167–198.

General Medical Council (1993). *Tomorrow's Doctors*. London: General Medical Council.

Giddens, A (1990). *The Problems of Modernity*. Cambridge: Polity Press.

Gillespie, R and C Gerhardt (1995). Social dimensions of sickness and disability. In Moon, G and R Gillespie (eds). *Society and Health*. London: Routledge, 79–96.

Gillon, R (1990). *Philosophical Medical Ethics*. Chichester: Wiley.

Gillon, R (1994). Medical ethics: four principles plus attention to scope. *British Medical Journal*, **309**, 184–188.

Giorgi, A (ed.) (1985). *Phenomenology and Psychological Research*. Pittsburgh: Duquesne University Press.

Glassner, B (1995). In the name of health. In Bunton, R, S Nettleton and R Burrows (eds). *The Sociology of Health Promotion: Critical Analyses of Consumption, Lifestyle and Risk*. London: Routledge, 159–173.

Glover, J (1999). *Humanity: A Moral History of the Twentieth Century*. London: Jonathan Cape.

Goffman, E (1961). *Asylums*. Harmondsworth: Penguin.

Habermas, J (1972). *Knowledge and Human Interests*. London: Heinemann.

Haldane, JJ (1986). 'Medical ethics'-an alternative approach. *Journal of Medical Ethics*, **12**, 145–150.

Halmos, P (1971). Sociology and the personal service professions. In Friedson, E (ed.) *The Professions and their Prospects*. Sage: Beverley Hills.

Hammersley, M and P Atkinson (1995). *Ethnography: Principles in Practice*. London: Routledge.

Hardey, M (1998). *The Social Context of Health*. Buckingham: Open University Press.

Hare, RM (1986). Health. *Journal of Medical Ethics*, **12**, 174–181.

Hart, C (2004). *Nurses and Politics: The Impact of Power and Practice*. Basingstoke: Palgrave-Macmillan.

Health Education Authority (1995). *Health and Lifestyles in the UK*. London: Health Eduation Authority.

Herzlich, C (1973). *Health and Illness*. New York: Academic Press.

Holliday, A (2002). *Doing and Writing Qualitative Research*. London: Sage.

Honey, P and A Mumford (1986). *The Manual of Learning Styles*. Maidenhead: Printique.

Howkins, EJ and A Ewens (1999). How students experience professional socialisation. *International Journal of Nursing Studies*, **35**, 41–49.

Howlett, B, WIU Ahmad and R Murray. An examination of Asian and Afro-Caribbean peoples' concepts of health and illness causation.

Paper presented at the *Annual Conference of the British Sociological Association*, Manchester, 25–28 March.

Hoyle, E (1980). Professionalisation and deprofessionalisation in education. In Hoyle, E and J Megarry (eds). *World Yearbook of Education 1980*. London: Kogan Page.

Illich, I (1975). *Medical Nemesis*. London: Calder and Boyars.

Illich, I (1977). *Limits to Medicine*. London: Pelican.

Illingworth, S (2004). *Approaches to Ethics in Higher Education: Teaching Ethics Across the Curriculum*. Leeds: PRS-LTSN.

Jones, I (2004). Using critical reflection in the paramedic curriculum. In Tate, S and M Sills (eds). *The Development of Critical Reflection in the Health Professions*. London: Higher Education Academy Health Sciences and Practice Subject Centre, 39–46.

Jones, L (1994). *The Social Context of Health and Health Work*. Basingstoke: Macmillan.

Jones, L (2000). What is health? In Katz, J, A Peberdy and J Douglas (eds). *Promoting Health: Knowledge and Practice* (Second Edition). Basingstoke: Palgrave, 18–36.

Jonsen, AR (1998). *The Birth of Bioethics*. Oxford: Oxford University Press.

Katz, J, A Peberdy and J Douglas (eds). (2001). *Promoting Health: Knowledge and Practice* (Second edition). Basingstoke: Palgrave.

Koehn, D (1994). *The Ground of Professional Ethics*. London: Routledge.

Kühn, TS (1962). *The Structure of Scientific Revolutions*. Chicago: University of Chicago Press.

Kühn, TS (1970). *The Structure of Scientific Revolutions* (Revised Edition). Chicago: University of Chicago Press.

Lacey, AR (1976). *A Dictionary of Philosophy*. London: Routledge and Kegan Paul.

Larson, MS (1977). *The Rise of Professionalism: A Sociological Analysis*. Berkeley, CA: University of California Press.

Lupton, D (1994). *Medicine as Culture*. London: Sage.

Lupton, D (1995). *The Imperative of Health: Public Health and the Regulated Body*. London: Sage.

Lupton, D (1996). *Food, the Body and the Self*. London: Sage.

McGuire, MB (1988). *Ritual Healing in Suburban United States*. New Brunswick: Rutgers University Press.

Macdonald, G and R Bunton (2002). Health promotion: disciplinary developments. In Bunton, R and G Macdonald (eds). *Health Promotion: Disciplines, Diversity and Developments* (Second Edition). London: Routledge, 9–28.

Magee, B (1975). *Popper*. London: Fontana.

Maibach, E and DA Murphy (1995). Self-efficacy in health promotion research and practice: conceptualization and measurement. *Health Education Research*, **10**, 1, 37–50.

Marshall, L and F Rowland (1998). *A Guide to Learning Independently* (Third Edition). Buckingham: Open University Press.

Marteau, TM (1990). Screening in practice: reducing the psychological costs. *British Medical Journal*, **301**, 26–28.

Melia, KM (1987). *Learning and Working: The Occupational Socialisation of Nurses*. London: Tavistock.

Merton, RK, GG Reader and PL Kendall (1957). *The Student Physician*. Cambridge, MA: Harvard University Press.

Mill, JS (1962). *Utilitarianism* (and other writings, ed. M Warnock). Glasgow: Fontana.

Morris, TV (1998). *If Aristotle Ran General Motors: The New Soul of Business*. New York: Henry Holt.

Mulhall, A (2001). Epidemiology. In Naidoo, J and J Wills (eds). *Health Studies: An Introduction*. Basingstoke: Palgrave, 39–68.

McKeown, T (1976). *The Role of Medicine: Dream, Mirage or Nemesis*. London: Nuffield Provincial Hospitals Trust.

Naidoo, J and J Wills (eds). (2001). *Health Studies: An Introduction*. Basingstoke: Palgrave.

O'Connor, A, A Hyde and M Treacy (2003). Nurse Teachers' construction of reflection and reflective practice. *Reflective Practice*, **4**, 2, 107–119.

Ogden, J (2001). Health psychology. In Naidoo, J and J Wills (eds). *Health Studies: An Introduction*. Basingstoke: Palgrave, 69–100.

Oxford University Press (1983). *The Oxford Paperback Dictionary* (Second Edition, compiled by Joyce M Hawkins). Oxford: Oxford University Press.

Paton, HJ (1948). *The Moral Law*. London: Hutchinson.

Peters, RS (1973). *Authority, Responsibility and Education* (Third Edition). London: George Allen and Unwin.

Pill, R and NCH Stott (1982). Concepts of illness causation and responsibility: Some preliminary data from a sample of working-class mothers. *Social Science and Medicine*, **16**, 1, 43–52.

Pill, R and NCH Stott (1985). Choice or chance: further evidence on ideas of illness and responsibility for health. *Social Science and Medicine*, **20**, 975–983.

Poppay, J and G. Williams (1994). *Researching the Peoples' Health*. London: Routledge.

Porter, S (1995). *Nursing's Relationship with Medicine: A Critical Realist Ethnography*. Aldershot: Avebury.

Powell, S (1999). *Returning to Study: A Guide for Professionals*. Buckingham: Open University Press.

Priest, V and V Speller (1991). *The Risk Factor Management Manual*. Oxford: Radcliffe Medical Press.

Prochaska, JO and CCD Diclemente (1982). Transtheoretical therapy: towards a more integrative model of change. *Psychotherapy: Theory, Research and Practice*, **19**, 276–288.

Quality Assurance Agency for Higher Education (2001). *Benchmark Statements for Health Care Programmes*. Gloucester: QAA.

Reich, WT (1995). *The Encyclopedia of Bioethics*. New York: Simon and Schuster-Macmillan.

Reid, DJ, AJ Killoran, AD McNeill and JS Chambers (1992). Choosing the most effective health promotion options for reducing a nation's smoking prevalence. *Tobacco Control*, 1, 185–197.

Rolfe, G, D Freshwater and M Jasper (2001). *Critical Reflection for Nursing and the Helping Professions: A User's Guide*. New York: Palgrave-Macmillan.

Roper, N (1976). *Clinical Experience in Nurse Education*.

Russsell, B (1979). *A History of Western Philosophy*. London: Unwin Paperbacks.

Scadding, JG (1988). Health and disease: what can medicine do for philosophy? *Journal of Medical Ethics*, 14, 118–124.

Scally, G and LJ Donaldson (1998). Clinical governance and the drive for quality improvement in the new NHS in England. *British Medical Journal*, 317, 61–65.

Scambler, G (2002). *Health and Social Change: A Critical Theory*. Buckingham: Open University Press.

Schön, D (1983). *The Reflective Practitioner*. New York: Basic Books.

Schön, D (1987). *Educating the Reflective Practitioner*. San Francisco, CA: Jossey-Bass.

Secretary of State for Health (1999). *Saving Lives: Our Healthier Nation*. London: The Stationery Office.

Seedhouse, D (1986). *Health: The Foundations for Achievement*. Chichester: Wiley.

Seedhouse, D (1988). *Ethics: The Heart of Health Care*. Chichester: Wiley.

Seedhouse, D (1995). 'Well-being': health promotion's red herring. *Health Promotion International*, 10, 1, 61–67.

Seedhouse, D (ed.) (1995). *Reforming Health Care: The Philosophy and Practice of International Health Reform*. Chichester: Wiley.

Seedhouse, D (1997). *Health Promotion: Philosophy, Prejudice and Practice*. Chichester: Wiley.

Seedhouse, D (2001). *Health: The Foundations for Achievement* (Second Edition). Chichester: Wiley.

Shweder, RA, NC Munch, M Mahapatra and L Park (1997). The 'big three' of morality (autonomy, community, divinity) and the 'big three' explanations of suffering. In Brandt, AM and P Rozin (eds). *Morality and Health*. New York: Routledge, 119–172.

Sider, RC and CD Clements (1984). Patients' ethical obligation for their health. *Journal of Medical Ethics*, 10, 138–142.

Skrabanek, P (1990). Why is preventive medicine exempt from ethical constraints? *Journal of Medical Ethics*, 16, 187–190.

Skrabanek, P and J McCormick (1989). *Follies and Fallacies in Medicine*. Glasgow: Tarragon Press.

Smith, WCS, MB Kenicer, A Maryon Davis, AE Evans and J Yarnell (1989). Blood cholesterol: is population screening warranted in the UK? *The Lancet*, 18 February, 372–373.

Sprague, E (1978). *Metaphysical Thinking*. New York: Oxford University Press.

Stephenson, A, R Higgs and J Sugarman (2001). Teaching professional development in medical schools. *The Lancet*, **357**, 867–870.

Stewart, R (1989). *Leading in the NHS*. Basingstoke: Macmillan.

Tate, S (2004). Using critical reflection as a teaching tool. In Tate, S and M Sills (eds). *The Development of Critical Reflection in the Health Professions*. London: Higher Education Academy Health Sciences and Practice Subject Centre, 8–17.

Tate, S and M Sills (eds). (2004). *The Development of Critical Reflection in the Health Professions*. London: Higher Education Academy Health Sciences and Practice Subject Centre.

Thorogood, N (2002). What is the relevance of sociology for health promotion? In Bunton, R and G Macdonald (eds). *Health Promotion: Disciplines, Diversity and Developments* (Second Edition). London: Routledge, 53–79.

Tilford, S, J Green and K Tones (2003). *Values, Health Promotion and the Public Health*. Leeds: Leeds Metropolitan University.

Tones, BK (1979). Past achievements, future successes. In Sutherland, I (ed.). *Health Education: Perspectives and Choices*. London: Allen and Unwin.

Tones, BK (1981). Affective education and health. In Cowley, J, K David and T Williams (eds). *Health Education in Schools*. London: Harper and Row.

Tones, BK and J Green (2004). *Health Promotion: Planning and Strategies*. London: Sage.

Turner, BS (2003). The history of the changing concepts of health and illness: outlines of a general model of illness categories. In Albrecht, GL, R Fitzpartick and S Scrimshaw (eds). *The Handbook of Social Studies in Health and Medicine*. London: Sage, 9–23.

United Kingdom Central Council for Nursing, Midwifery and Health Visiting (1986). *Project 2000: A New Preparation for Practice*. London: UKCC.

University of Auckland (1993). *Managing Postgraduate Research Students*. Auckland: University of Auckland.

Urmson, JO (1967). The interpretation of the moral philosophy of JS Mill. In Foot, P (ed.). *Theories of Ethics*. Oxford: Oxford University Press, 128–136.

Webster, C and J French (2002). The cycle of conflict: the history of the public health and health promotion movements. In Adams, L,

M Amos and J Munro (eds). *Promoting Health: Politics and Practice*. London: Sage.

White, P (2004). Using reflective practice in the physiotherapy curriculum. In Tate, S and M Sills (eds). *The Development of Critical Reflection in the Health Professions*. London: Higher Education Academy Health Sciences and Practice Subject Centre, 24–31.

Wikler, D (1987). Who should be blamed for being sick? *Health Education Quarterly*, **14**, 1, 11–25.

Williams, R (1983). Concepts of health: an analysis of lay logic. *Sociology*, **17**, 2, 185–204.

Williams, SJ (2003). *Medicine and the Body*. London: Sage.

Wilkinson, R (1996). *Unhealthy Societies: The Afflictions of Inequality*. London: Routledge.

Wilson, M (1975). *Health is for People*. London: Darton, Longman and Todd.

Wilson-Barnett, J and J Macleod-Clark (1993). From sick nursing to health nursing; evolution or revolution? In Wilson-Barnett, J and J Macleod-Clark (eds). *Research in Health Promotion and Nursing*. Basingstoke: Macmillan, 256–270.

World Health Organisation (1946). *Constitution*. WHO: New York.

Wörner, M (2000). Elements of an ethics of health promotion. *First International Conference on Ethics, Politics and Health Promotion*, Cavan, Republic of Ireland (17–19 April).

Young, M (2004). Using reflective practice in the podiatry curriculum. In Tate, S and M Sills (eds). *The Development of Critical Reflection in the Health Professions*. London: Higher Education Academy Health Sciences and Practice Subject Centre, 18–23.

Zola, IK (1972). Medicine as an institution of social control. *Sociological Review*, **20**, 487–503.

Index